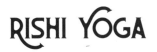

RISHI YOGA

Movement Meditation Practices
of the Himalayan Sages

PIERRE BONNASSE

Translated by Karina Bharucha

Inner Traditions
Rochester, Vermont

Inner Traditions
One Park Street
Rochester, Vermont 05767
www.InnerTraditions.com

Originally published in 2017 in French under the title *Rishi-yoga: La méditation dynamique de l'Himalaya* by Éditions Dervy, 19 rue Saint-Séverin, 75005 Paris
First U.S. edition published in 2019 by Inner Traditions

Note to the reader: *This book is intended as an informational guide. The remedies, approaches, and techniques described herein are meant to supplement, and not to be a substitute for, professional medical care or treatment. They should not be used to treat a serious ailment without prior consultation with a qualified health care professional.*

Cataloging-in-Publication Data for this title is available from the Library of Congress

ISBN 978-1-62055-786-0 (print)
ISBN 978-1-62055-787-7 (ebook)

Printed and bound in the United States by Versa Press, Inc.

10 9 8 7 6 5 4 3 2 1

Text design and layout by Priscilla Baker
This book was typeset in Garamond Premier Pro with Besitoea, Avant Garde, and Gill Sans used as display typefaces

To send correspondence to the author of this book, mail a first-class letter to the author c/o Inner Traditions • Bear & Company, One Park Street, Rochester, VT 05767, and we will forward the communication, or contact the author directly at **www.nidra-yoga.com.**

Contents

Introduction   1

PART I
BASICS
Practicing Rishi Yoga Meditation

PART II
EXPLORATION
Complementary Practices

PART III
REFLECTION
Philosophical Perspectives

Introduction

The Rishi Yoga Meditation is a practice comprised of easy physical poses and movements, aided by an appropriate inner attitude, and logically combined with breathing exercises, sensory listening, and concentration, allowing for the very nature of meditation and contemplation to reveal itself in a simple and natural way, at the heart of ordinary movements and actions of daily life.

Based on simple principles that are applicable by everyone, this ancestral practice, transmitted by Himalayan yogis, draws its strength from its simplicity and a variety of exercises, as well as from its inventiveness, and numerous possibilities of adaptation to a wide field of application. This is how, after having spent some time in the Himalayas, Alfonso Caycedo created "sophrology"* and its twelve "dynamic

---

*According to Wikipedia, the term Sophrology comes from ancient Greek *sôs* (healthy), *phrēn* (mind), and *-logia* (study of), and is a personal development technique founded in 1960 by Alfonso Caycedo, a Colombian neuropsychiatrist. It studies individual consciousness in order to allow a more conscious living. The term Sophrology has never been protected in its public use and resulted in many variations and divergences. Caycedo registered his original discipline as "Caycedian Sophrology." Sophrology in everyday use can refer either to Caycedian Sophrology or to other derived forms.

During his research, Caycedo was guided by various traditions and currents, both Eastern and Western. Among the most influential for Sophrology were hypnosis and phenomenology, as well as yoga and Buddhism, mainly Zen Buddhism.

Sophrology has its own methodology and original techniques, aiming to develop awareness in daily life and the autonomy of those who practice it. It is widely practiced in France today. —Trans.

relaxation" techniques in the sixties. Even though sophrology has its own jargon, approach, and methodology, in its essence it is clearly and considerably inspired by ancient yoga practices, and most probably by this little-known practice that summarizes everything by refocusing on its main aim.

In Indian philosophy, regardless of the points of view, this aim has always been the recognition of the Divine, whose nature is described as "Being-Consciousness-Bliss." Being omnipresent, this nature is neither external nor internal, neither material nor spiritual, but it is present as the common essence of all phenomena and all beings. Multiple forms appear in the Oneness and dissolve in the Oneness itself.

In the same manner, if the essence of all phenomena is always Consciousness or Awareness, which this process invites us to probe so that it reveals itself, the practices attempting to access it are numerous, and can be adapted in an infinite number of ways. This is why the form and its adaptations proposed in this book, although transmitted in a traditional context, are just a suggestion among others, far from any kind of dogmatism or sectarianism; one can assimilate and adapt them according to one's understanding, needs, and objectives.

Here, conceiving and retaining a rigid method in an intellectual way for developing a new kind of therapy is not important. The main aim is to offer simple tools that promote the well-being of the body and the mind, and to especially allow one to open up to the essential dimension of one's being, beyond name and form, from which one can subsequently discern the numerous possibilities that can be freely explored.

The Dynamic Meditation described here constitutes a foundation for all variations or adaptations that can be done. Firstly, it allows one to stimulate, align, and recognize the fundamental structures of the being, through which the actions of the body and the mind take place. With progressive logic, the alert perception of these structures subsequently allows for the awakening to the unconscious dimension of the being, which ultimately reveals the Awareness itself, the unchanging witness of all phenomena, experiences, and states. But this essential realization does not necessarily involve any kind of progression or evolution: it can happen at any time, and through any bodily or mental action or movement. That being said, progressive logic allows for the recognition of the structures of the being, inextricably linked with the so-called states of Awareness, according to a process that goes from the most gross to the most subtle, and that can lead to the revelation of this light of Awareness that illuminates the process itself.

Thus, this basic approach will first allow for the awareness of the physical body and its tissues (skin, muscles, bones, and organs), focusing especially on the glands, joints, and spine, in order to warm up and deeply relax the central nervous system, through which the circulation of the vital life energy can be intimately felt. Indeed, the body is composed of meridians or energy channels, the most important of which are located in the spine. The crossing point of channels constitutes an energy center that stores and distributes the energy. The spine is therefore the abode of six important energy centers, which are all connected to other centers mainly located in the joints of the body where numerous channels cross over, and which ensure the distribution of the vital energy throughout the body. When blocks or knots form at these junctions, it obstructs the flow of energy, and can cause physical and mental disorders. In this way, through simple movements such as applying pressure, bending, stretching, and rotating, further reinforced by the alert synchronization of the breath, this basic Dynamic Meditation will allow for maintaining and restoring the correct flow of vital energy in the entire body, all the while favoring a better awareness of physical, energetic, and mental phenomena.

The attentive perceiving of these phenomena allows for the revelation of the very space of attention in which they arise. Gradually, the frontier between the conscious and the unconscious begins to give way, until the light illuminating all processes is fully revealed. And then comes the discovery of everlasting peace, pure Awareness, ever-present joy of being, and the revelation that all this has always been here, regardless of the place, the time, or the circumstances. This essential recognition of the Self, of the essence of being, allows us to instantly realize that our true nature is free of everything that appears and disappears in it. By intimately understanding that the witness of physical, respiratory, and mental movements does not move, that the witness of any kind of tension is without tension, and that the witness of suffering does not suffer, one can be free of what one believes oneself to be. Thus, a new dimension of existence opens up. Even if nothing changes in the external aspects of one's life, this life will nevertheless emerge in a silent space, overflowing with joy, always calm and peaceful, in which even the strongest and most concealed emotions will eventually manifest, and then fade away.

PART I
BASICS

Practicing Rishi Yoga
Meditation

General Instructions
for Rishi Yoga Meditation

Rishi Yoga Meditation lends itself to many variations, and can be adapted and adjusted in endless ways, depending on the needs of the moment. It is possible to do the full version composed of 108 exercises or shorten and adapt it to suit one's needs.* One can practice as often as one likes and for as long as one likes. Many of the steps of the exercises lend themselves to being done either while standing up, in a sitting position on a chair or the floor, or lying down, according to one's requirements and abilities and according to the context. Anything is possible, as long as the exercises are performed logically, consistently, in a balanced and gentle manner, and with full awareness. In this way, the practice and its numerous possible alternatives allow for a detailed and deep exploration of the structures of the being, with varying degrees of progress.

Although on the surface this series of exercises seems to be a

---

*The number 108 has been long considered a sacred number in traditions like Hinduism, Buddhism, and Jainism as well as in yoga. The number's significance is open to interpretation. Some believe that renowned Vedic mathematicians viewed 108 as a number of the wholeness of existence. Others say that this number connects the sun, the moon, and the Earth, because the average distance of the sun and the moon to the Earth is 108 times their respective diameters. According to yogic tradition, there are 108 *pithas* or sacred sites throughout India, 108 Upanishads, and 108 *marmas* or sacred regions in the body.

sequence of movements performed by the body, it does not in the least constitute a gymnastic exercise. Even if it is possible to accelerate the movements from time to time, they are generally performed slowly, and always with full awareness of the body and the breath, with consistent attention to sensations, emotions, thoughts, images, and all phenomena that appear and disappear in the peaceful, silent, and still space of Awareness, which the attentive perception of the moment and other phenomena reveals naturally. The attitude must be one of welcoming, listening, and openness, without effort or grasping, accepting everything that manifests with equanimity and attention.

This has nothing to do with a proactive or deliberate attitude, grounded in the belief of being someone who is doing, accessing, attaining, or succeeding in doing something. True surrender is to simply let go of the one who is holding onto something (or believes that he or she is holding onto something), more than letting go of what is being held. Therefore, the exercises should be regularly interspersed with breaks (sitting down or standing up, according to the choice of the practitioner, as long as the position is stable and comfortable) during which one is advised to abandon oneself and recognize oneself in the silent space of Awareness, in which the movement will unfold and subsequently subside, without identifying with the energy of the movement and the phenomena. The clouds are moving, but the sky remains undisturbed and free of everything that is happening in it.

To Begin

1. Seated (on a chair or on the floor) or standing up, start by being aware of the silent space in which sounds appear and disappear. Do not try to change anything, just be aware of the general state of your body and of your breath in this eternal and naturally present silence.

2. Observe your natural breathing for a few moments, and then become aware of your body, part by part, while observing your breath.

* First, be aware of your head, on the surface and then inside.
* Then, your neck.
* Then, your shoulders, arms, chest, sides, and upper back.
* Then, the abdominal and lumbar belts.
* Then, the sacral and sexual regions.
* From the anus to the tip of your toes.
* Lastly, be aware of the entire body breathing in the silent space.

During these seven steps, do not try to relax your body, but feel how this relaxation occurs naturally and spontaneously, as a result of being aware and of being in contact with the silence. At every stage, simply notice all phenomena (sensations, emotions, thoughts, or images) appearing and disappearing in the silent space.

3. If physical or mental tension persists, particularly if the mind is agitated, note that the silent space in which this tension and this agitation appear is neither tensed nor agitated. Observe that these tensions or this agitation are naturally surrounded by a tranquil silence. Breathe in, hold your breath for a few seconds, and become aware of this silence in which the agitation has just dissolved, then exhale slowly. Repeat this twice or thrice if necessary. Notice the presence of the silent space in the body and all around. Everything appears and disappears in it.

4. Chant the mantra *OM* (*AUM*) by inhaling deeply, and chanting with the longest exhale possible, while being aware of the vibrations of the sound in your whole body and in the surrounding space. Observe that the sound emerges from and dissolves in the silence, and that this silence is always present with the sound, like a backdrop. Then, stay immersed in this silence.

5. Continue breathing deeply. While inhaling, become aware of the energy (sound, light, vibration) in the center of your head, between the eyebrows. While exhaling, feel the subtle movement of the expansion of this energy in the entire head region, and in the surrounding space.

* With every breath, notice that the presence of the body, of the vital energy, and of the joy of being becomes more and more sensitive and obvious. Observe that this is not the result of some personal action, but of a listening that is developing, and of an opening that is revealing itself naturally.

* Then allow this listening to spread to the cervical, dorsal, lumbar, sacral, and coccygeal regions, and to the whole spine.

* As you inhale, be aware of the energy field in a specific region of the body; and as you exhale, be aware of its gentle expansion in the entire organic structure, along with the uninterrupted joy of being

that emerges and fills up the entire space, thus infusing every cell of the body.

* Observe all phenomena that appear in the Awareness: the sensations, emotions, thoughts, images, sounds, and silences. Notice that Awareness is there, but there is nobody to be aware of it. Acknowledge that "me," "I," or "I am doing" are also thoughts appearing and disappearing in Awareness; and that the space of consciousness and of silent welcoming is naturally present, even before any kind of claim about accomplishing an action arises.

* Allow the rest of the Dynamic Meditation to happen spontaneously in this silent space of the witness untouched by all that is taking place automatically.

Exercises for the Cranial Center

6. Place both hands on your head and notice its shape, texture, presence, and how it feels. Is the Awareness inside your head, or is your head appearing in the space of Awareness? Observe the phenomena that appear in the silent space, for the duration of the entire practice.

7. Be aware of the vital energy in your hands and in your fingertips, and then massage your scalp vigorously. Then let your arms hang loosely alongside your body (if you are standing) or place them on your thighs or knees (if you are sitting).

8. Inhale and pucker your forehead, as if you are frowning; relax it as you exhale. Then inhale, hold your breath, and rapidly pucker and relax your forehead, several times. Finally, relax your forehead as you exhale with full awareness of all phenomena that appear and disappear in the space of consciousness. Do this several times, according to time available and as much as you need to.

9. Massage your forehead with your thumbs, moving from the middle of your forehead toward the temples.

10. Massage your temples with your index and middle fingers, with clockwise and counterclockwise circular movements.

11. Gently pinch your eyebrows with your thumbs and index fingers, and massage them gently, from the center toward the ends.

12. Massage your sinuses with the sides of your index fingers, by rubbing them with a downward movement.

13. Do the following eye movements: from left to right and right to left; up and down; diagonally, from top right to bottom left, then from top left to bottom right; look at all four corners, as if you are drawing a square; do circular eye movements, clockwise and counterclockwise; blink several times; inhale, close your eyelids tightly, then exhale and relax.

14. With your arms stretched out in front of you at shoulder height and your elbows straight, bring both thumbs up; move your right thumb to the right, your left thumb to the left, and look at both thumbs simultaneously. Bring them together and move them apart. Repeat this a few times.

15. With your arms stretched out in front of you at shoulder height and your elbows straight, bring both thumbs up. Stare at your thumbs without blinking, until tears appear. Close your eyes and observe.

16. Look at the tip of your nose without blinking.

17. Rub your palms together until they become warm and then place them on your eyes, and feel the warmth and the darkness.

18. Tighten and relax one cheek after the other, and then both cheeks simultaneously; and finally, your whole face.

19. Massage your nose with your palm.

20. Tighten and relax your nose.

21. Massage your jaws by placing your palms on your cheeks, and applying gentle pressure as you slowly move your palms up and down.

22. Pull your earlobes down, then pull your ears sideways, then turn and twist them.

23. Close your eyes with your index fingers, move your fingers gently, and then remove them.

24. Close your ears with your hands and listen to the sound coming from inside your body.

25. Massage your ears.

26. Tighten and relax your ears.

27. Open and close your mouth.

28. Chew.

29. Close your mouth, fill it with air for a while, and then churn or gargle the air.

30. Stick your tongue out as far as possible and roar like a lion.

31. Move your jaws from right to left, left to right, and up and down.

32. Clench your teeth tightly, and then make a sound by gently banging your teeth against each other.

33. Tighten and relax one side of your face, then the other side, both sides, and finally, your whole face.

34. Rub your hands together and massage your head and face.

35. Seated or standing up, pause for a moment in order to become aware of the sensations or vibrations in your whole head, as they appear. Be aware of them, feel them, allow your attention to touch the skin of your face and skull, your nose, mouth (and tongue), and your eyes; feel all five sense organs simultaneously, and be aware of all phenomena that emerge and subside. Then, inhale with full awareness of the vital energy from the eyebrow center and mentally repeat "I"; exhale with awareness of the expansion of the energy in your whole head (skin, muscles, organs, and bones) and in the space all around, and mentally repeat "Am," as you enjoy the joy of being in all your cells and in the silent space.

Exercises for the Cervical Center

36. Place your hands on your neck and notice its shape, texture, presence, and how it feels. Feel the presence of your neck in the silent space.

37. Inhale, hold your breath, tighten your chin and the front part of your neck as you clench your teeth, and then exhale completely. Repeat this several times. Feel what happens. Observe the sensations.

38. Open your mouth, place your index, middle, and ring fingers in your mouth, down your throat, and chant "aaaaaa" three times. Feel the expansion of the vibration in space.

39. Raise your shoulders to your ears as you inhale, and lower them as you exhale. Feel your trapezius muscles. Repeat this several times, in sync with your breath. Then, do it several times as you hold your breath. Feel the pull of gravity.

40. Place your fingertips on your shoulders; turn your torso to the left, and then to the right several times. Rotate your shoulders forward and backward.

41. Let your arms hang loosely alongside your body and rotate your shoulders in one direction and then in the opposite direction. Observe the sensations at the base of your neck.

42. Move your head and neck up and down, as if you are saying "yes": exhale when your chin touches your chest and inhale when your chin moves upward. You can do this again, as you hold your breath in or with empty lungs. Feel the movement of the energy when your chin is against your chest.

43. Move your head from the right to left, and then from the left to right, as if you are saying "no." Repeat as indicated above.

44. Move your head forward like a turtle as you exhale, and pull it back as you inhale. Repeat a few times.

45. Move your head sideways, as if you want to touch your ear to your shoulder. In order to increase the neck stretch, when the right ear is on the right shoulder, place your right hand on the top of your head and press your head down gently. Repeat the exercise on the left side.

46. Do circular head movements in one direction and then in the opposite direction. Do this exercise several times, in sync with your breath; then do it again as you hold your breath. Ask yourself: "Who is moving during the exercise? Am I moving or am I still? Am I moving my head, or am I the still spectator of a head moving in 'me,' in the silent space that I am?" Observe this.

47. Rub your palms together until they are warm, and then gently massage your neck; be aware of its shape, presence, and of the different sensations.

48. Seated or standing up, pause for a moment in order to become aware of the sensations or vibrations in your whole neck, as they appear. Then, inhale with full awareness of the vital energy from the cervical center (in the cervical spine) and mentally repeat "I"; exhale with the awareness of the expansion of the energy in your whole neck (skin, muscles, organs, and bones) and in the surrounding space, and mentally repeat "Am," as you enjoy the joy of being in all your cells and in the silent space.

Exercises for the Dorsal Center
and the Arms

49. Place your hands on your sternum, and notice its shape, its presence, and how it feels. Feel the presence of the upper part of your torso and your arms in the silent space.

50. Place your fists in front of your sternum, open the chest cavity as you inhale, pulling your elbows back; then exhale and relax. Let your body and mind expand in the conscious space as you inhale. Repeat a few times.

51. Stretch your arms out to the sides; make small circles, and then big circles, in one direction, and then the opposite direction. Then make the circles smaller, without getting carried away by the energy of the movement, and welcome it in the silent and still space that does not move. With your arms outstretched, stay still as the space, as the witness of the moving body. Repeat several times.

52. With your arms still stretched out to the sides, inhale and open them wider by pulling them back; then exhale and bring your outstretched arms to the front. Do this several times.

53. With your arms stretched out to the sides, inhale and bring your hands to your shoulders, palms facing down; exhale and extend your arms to the front at shoulder height; inhale and bring your hands to your chest, and then exhale and raise your arms overhead; inhale and bring your hands to your shoulders; exhale and hold your arms wide apart. Repeat the full sequence. Feel the movement coming from the emptiness.

54. Place your hands on your shoulders with your arms parallel to the ground, then extend your arms in front of you at shoulder height; bring your hands back to your shoulders, then extend and stretch them out sideways, then bring them back to your shoulders. Do this several times with full awareness of the movement at the elbow level.

55. With interlocked hands, rotate your wrists in one direction and then in the opposite direction.

56. Rotate your hands in both directions, and then move them up and down, to the right and the left. Make your hands into claws and rotate them; then make them into fists and rotate them. Repeat several times.

57. Open and close your hands and fingers in a rapid manner.

58. With your arms stretched outward, tighten your fists, then bring them to your chest, as if you are pulling on a cord.

59. Massage your hands and the joints of each finger; interlock and stretch your fingers by extending your arms in front of you.

60. Seated or standing up, pause for a moment in order to become aware of the sensations and vibrations in your chest, back, and arms as they appear. Then, inhale with full awareness of the vital energy from the dorsal center (in the thoracic spine between the shoulder blades) and mentally repeat "I"; exhale with full awareness of the expansion of energy in your chest (skin, muscles, organs, and bones) and in the surrounding space, and mentally repeat "Am" as you enjoy the joy of being in all your cells and in the silent space. Feel the heart (the organ) beat in the still, silent, and formless space of the (spiritual) Heart. Stay there, in the here and now. Who am I? Who can see? To whom do the answers appear?

Exercises for the Lumbar Center

61. Place your hands on your navel and notice the form of your belly, its presence, your breath and touch.

62. Allow the abdominal zone to swell as you breathe in, and let it deflate as you exhale; do this rapidly, then slowly, then rapidly again, and so on. Repeat several times.

63. Practice the "breath of fire," inhaling and exhaling through your nose forcefully and rhythmically with your belly engaged.

 * After several breaths, inhale and hold your breath, then exhale completely through your mouth as you bend forward, with your back straight, your tongue sticking out, and your hands on your thighs.
 * Then, without inhaling, suck your tummy inward and upward, and "churn the fire" by rapidly pulling in your belly and pushing it out, in order to massage your internal organs and increase body heat; then suck your belly in for a few seconds, and hold it in.
 * Straighten up slowly, push your belly out, and inhale gently as your body straightens completely. Observe the natural breath and the movement of the energy from your abdomen. Feel the heat and energy spread to your whole body.

64. Make your hands into claws and, as you inhale, bend backward slightly, as if you are trying to support a heavy weight, contracting the abdominal wall powerfully as you hold your breath; then let go as you exhale and straighten your body. Observe the natural abdominal breathing and the movement of the diaphragm massaging the solar plexus.

65. Seated or standing up, pause for a moment in order to notice the sensations and vibrations in the entire abdominal and lumbar regions as they appear.

* Then, inhale with full awareness of the vital energy from the lumbar center (level with the navel) and mentally repeat "I."

* Exhale with the awareness of the expansion of energy in your whole belly (skin, muscles, organs, and bones), in the solar plexus, and all around (in space), and mentally repeat "Am," as you enjoy the joy of being in all your cells and in the silent space.

* Feel the physical body's gravity center (two fingers below the belly-button) and the feeling of terrestrial gravity appearing in the silent space of Awareness, which is neither heavy nor light. Stay there, in the here and now.

Exercises for the Sacral Center

66. Place one hand on your lower abdomen and the other one on the sacral region, and notice their shape, presence, and touch.

67. Stand up and place your hands on your hips; move your pelvis forward and backward, then from left to right, and finally in a circular manner in both directions.

68. With your arms hanging loosely alongside your body, turn to one side and then to the other, rotating around the central axis.

69. Standing on one leg, hold your other knee with one hand; bring it to your chest, and push your leg to the side. Bring it back to the center and push it sideways again, balancing on one leg. Reverse legs and repeat.

70. Sit with your back straight and legs stretched out. Place one foot on the inner side of the opposite arm, at elbow level, and hold your bent leg by hugging it with both arms, with fingers interlocked for a firm grip. Move your leg from left to right and right to left ("rock the baby"); then, without letting go, bring your foot to your chest as you exhale completely (the other leg remains stretched out). Do this exercise with both legs and remain aware of your hips as they open up.

71. Be seated with your back straight and place your heels against the perineum; hold the soles of both feet together with your hands.

* Raise both knees as you inhale, and lower them as you exhale, several times.

* Then inhale deeply, and let your upper body bend forward as you exhale, starting with the sexual region, the lower abdomen, the belly, and so on, as if you want your forehead to touch the floor.

* Move down with each exhaling breath and let gravity operate. Do not strain by focusing on the resistance of the tendons and bones. Feel the empty space in your hips and allow the movement to happen on its own in this emptiness. Explore, without strain or effort.

72. Inhale, firmly contract the sexual region (sexual organs and perineum), and hold your breath for a few moments; then exhale and let go. Become aware of the energy rising in the emptiness.

73. Seated or standing up, pause for a moment in order to notice the sensations and vibrations in the sexual and sacral regions as they appear.

* Then, inhale with awareness of the vital energy from the sacral center (level with the sacrum) and mentally repeat "I."

* Exhale with the awareness of the entire sexual region (skin, muscles, organs, and bones) and the surrounding space, and mentally repeat "Am," as you enjoy the joy of being in all your cells and in the silent space.

* Then, inhaling, pull the energy in the spine upward, to the top of your head, and let it fall back down as you exhale. Feel the ebb and flow of the vibrations that appear and disappear in the silent and empty space.

Exercises for the Coccyx Center
and the Legs

74. Place your hands on your thighs and notice their shape, presence, and touch.

75. Tighten your anus (external sphincter) in a powerful way as you inhale, and relax as you exhale. Contract and relax in the same manner while holding your breath with full or empty lungs, keep your attention open to the movement of the energy in the spine during the phases of inhaling and contracting. Repeat a few times.

76. Contract your anus in a powerful way; keep the external sphincter clenched, then contract and relax the internal sphincter (rectum), and finally, relax completely. Remain attentive to the energy rising in the spine.

77. Stand up, bend forward from your waist, place your hands on your knees, bend them in order to bring your buttocks to your heels, and then stand up again by straightening your legs and keeping your back straight; synchronize the movement with your breath. Repeat several times.

78. With your legs slightly flexed, feet placed together, and your hands on your knees, do circular knee movements, from left to right and right to left; and then, inward to outward and outward to inward. Straighten your legs and use your hands to gently rotate your kneecaps. Repeat several times.

79. Raise one leg slightly as you balance on the other one, and activate your ankle by moving your foot up and down, sideways (from left to right), and in circles in both directions. Do the same with your other leg.

80. Move your toes up and down; then, keep your big toe up and push the others down, and finally, the other way around.

81. Place your toes on the ground and make circles with your feet.

82. Walk and jump in place (on the spot).

83. Bend one leg then the other, alternately kicking each side of your buttocks with the heel of your bent leg. Repeat several times.

84. Shake each relaxed leg, one after the other.

85. Once again, tighten and loosen the anus several times, as you suck the energy upward in the spine.

86. Seated or standing up, pause for a moment and notice the sensations and vibrations in the entire anal region and in your legs, all the way down to your toes, as they appear.

* Then, inhale with awareness of the vital energy from the coccyx center (level with the tailbone) and mentally repeat "I"; exhale with awareness of the entire anal region, of your legs (skin, muscles, organs, and bones) and the surrounding space, and mentally repeat "Am," as you enjoy the joy of being in all your cells and in the silent space.

* Then, pull the energy in the spine upward to the top of your head, and let it fall back down as you exhale. Feel the ebb and flow of the vibrations that appear and disappear in the silent and empty space.

Exercises for the Spine
(and All Centers)

87. Let your arms dangle alongside your body and notice their shape and presence, and the verticality of the body in the silent space. Feel the sensation of the whole body appearing in awareness. Feel the awareness in the body and all around, effortlessly.

88. Keeping your hands level with the lower abdomen, interlock your fingers, inhale, and push your palms up toward the sky; hold your breath, feel your whole body and the space all around; push the ground with the soles of your feet and push the sky with your palms, stretching your spine as much as possible; exhale and bring both arms down alongside your body. Repeat a few times.

89. Inhale and raise your hands and palms to the sky, stretch your body, exhale and bend your upper body sideways to the right; inhale as you come back to the center and exhale as you bend your body sideways to the left; then inhale as you come back to the center once again, and bring your arms back down. Repeat a few times.

90. Inhale as you raise your arms and push them backward; exhale as you allow your relaxed upper body to bend forward, keeping your legs straight. Feel the spine floating in the void. Hold the pose for a few breaths.

91. Rotate the trunk by making circular movements with your upper body, as you stretch the spine. Repeat a few times.

92. Keeping your arms, legs, and back straight, interlock your fingers behind your back and bend forward to touch your head to your knees, and take several breaths. Then, bend your knees as much as possible, with your belly on your thighs, and bring your arms over your head; release the tension in the hands, arms, and head, and breathe deeply.

93. Contract and relax each side of your body, then both sides simultaneously (your whole body): inhale, raise one arm straight up toward the sky and balance your body weight on the leg on the same side as the raised arm; hold your breath, keeping your arm raised, and feel the contraction of half your body (and your raised arm) in the emptiness, while the other half remains relaxed. Exhale and come back to the initial position. Repeat the exercise on the other side, and then with both arms and both sides of the body contracted.

94. Legs apart and arms open wide to the sides:
* Inhale in the still center, exhale as you bend to the right and place your right hand on your right foot. Look at your left hand pointing to the sky, stay with empty lungs and listen to the silent space.
* Inhale and come back to the center and repeat the exercise on the opposite side as you exhale.
* During the whole exercise, feel the "wheel" turning in one direction and then the other, from the empty and still center. The wheel turns in the empty space, which is untouched by the wheel and by the movement. Repeat a few times.

95. Keep your feet shoulder-width apart and your arms alongside your body, fists clenched:
* Inhale and raise your arms to the sky; exhale and bring them down as you place your buttocks near your heels, with your back straight.

* Then inhale, as you come up again and raise your arms; exhale as you go back down, and so on.
* Repeat this several times with forceful breathing. Take a little time to rest in the center, as you welcome the phenomena.

96. Shake your whole body with rapid, jerky movements, keeping your heels firmly stuck to the ground, and your muscles completely relaxed, all the while trying to maintain a slight tightening of the anus. Then, inhale, hold your breath, contract the anus powerfully as you suck the energy upward, and relax completely as you exhale. Feel the warmth, light, and vibration spreading in the silent space. Enjoy the feeling. Do this for several seconds.

97. Sit cross-legged on the floor or on a chair:
* Hold on to your right knee with your left hand, twist your right arm behind your back; inhale in the center, push the top of your head gently upward and your perineum to the ground.
* Exhale slowly and deeply with your back straight as you turn your chest, shoulders, and head to the right, and look behind. Stay still in this position and breathe deeply as you observe the breath passing through your left nostril.
* Come back to the center, synchronizing the movement with your breath; relax the whole body completely.
* Then repeat the exercise on the other side (ensuring that you observe the breath passing through your right nostril).
* Come back to the center, observe the breath coming and going through both nostrils simultaneously.

98. In the same position, with your back straight, hold your right wrist with your left hand behind your back, level with the sacral region:
* Inhale as you suck the energy upward in your spine, up to the empty space above your head.

* Exhale and allow the upper body to bend forward, lowering your lower abdomen onto your thighs, then lowering your belly, chest, and finally your forehead to the floor, or as far down as possible, as you observe the energy descending into the empty space under the tailbone. Breathe into the spine for a few moments in this position, and feel the breath and energy come and go in the silent space.

99. Lying on your back, practice the "crocodile series" for the flexibility of the whole spine:

* Extend your arms out to your sides, place your right foot on your left foot as you inhale; then exhale and turn your feet to the right and your head to the left. Do this on the other side with feet reversed.

* Do the same exercise with your feet crossed, one ankle placed on the other, and repeat with feet reversed.

* Then, do it with one foot at the level of the other knee, and repeat with feet reversed.

* Do it with your heels near your buttocks and feet apart and then with your heels, buttocks, and feet touching.

* Then do it with your knees on your chest: wrap your arms around your knees and bring your head to your knees, in a cowering position. Breathe deeply.

* Relax and lie down on your back, with your arms and legs spread out slightly. Observe the rise and fall of the breath in the spine, and surrender to the profound and silent tranquility in the background, to the silent and still space in which the rising and falling appear and disappear.

Deep Relaxation and "Conscious Sleep" (Yoga Nidra)

100. *Preparation:*

* Lie down on your back, with your spine, neck, and head properly aligned, your arms and legs slightly apart, eyes closed, your palms turned upward or toward the floor, and become aware of this stable and comfortable posture called the "corpse pose" or "dead body pose."

* Notice the body, the breath, gravitational pull, and the different points of support, effortlessly: there is nothing to do, nothing to make up, create, imagine, gain, attain, expect, or desire; simply recognize what is already there by being aware of the general state of the body and mind, without trying to change anything. Do not name anything; just welcome the phenomena that appear and disappear in the conscious tranquility, like clouds in the sky. Remain simply in the here and now, without form or intention. Just be.

101. *Conscious relaxation:*

* By remaining in the witness "state," attentive and balanced in the face of all sensations that arise in the silent space, become aware of your body from the top of your head to the tips of your

toes, and from your toes to the top of your head in the following sequence:

* Top of the head, scalp, forehead, temples, eyebrows, eyelids, eyes, eyeballs, nostrils, cheeks, lips, mouth, tongue, chin, neck, back of the neck, throat, shoulders, upper arms, elbows, forearms, wrists, back of your hands, palms, fingers up to your fingertips, and then once again from the fingertips up to the elbows.

* Then, your armpits, chest, back, ribs, sides, lower back, belly, lower abdomen, sacral region, hips, buttocks, perineum, thighs, knees, calves, shins, ankles, and the feet from the heels to the toes.

* Then come back to the initial point, being aware of all the points from your toes to the top of your head.

* For a few minutes, effortlessly observe the sensations from the top of your head to your toes while exhaling, and from your toes to the top of your head while inhaling. Be the detached observer of the wave of breath that rises and falls freely with natural breathing. Feel that the wave comes and goes in the space of Awareness, without any tension, naturally still and silent.

102. *Journey in the body:*

* Place your attention in a point in the center of your head (point 1), and feel the ebb and flow of the vibrations radiating from this point or field, with every inhaling and exhaling breath. Feel it spread to the organs, flesh, and bones, to the skin, and to the space all around. Be aware of the sixty-one key points in the following order, taking the time to feel each point, for two or three breaths.

1. Center of the head
2. Throat
3. Right shoulder joint
4. Elbow
5. Wrist
6. Tip of the right thumb
7. Tip of the index finger
8. Tip of the middle finger
9. Tip of the ring finger
10. Tip of the little finger
11. Right wrist joint
12. Elbow
13. Right shoulder joint
14. Throat
15. Left shoulder joint
16. Elbow
17. Wrist
18. Tip of the left thumb
19. Tip of the index finger
20. Tip of the middle finger
21. Tip of the ring finger
22. Tip of the little finger
23. Left wrist joint
24. Elbow
25. Left shoulder joint
26. Throat
27. Center of the chest (heart)
28. Right side of the chest
29. Center of the chest (heart)
30. Left side of the chest
31. Center of the chest (heart)
32. Navel
33. Lower abdomen
34. Right hip
35. Knee
36. Right ankle
37. Tip of the right big toe
38. Tip of the second toe
39. Tip of the third toe
40. Tip of the fourth toe
41. Tip of the little toe
42. Right ankle
43. Knee
44. Hip
45. Lower abdomen
46. Left hip
47. Knee
48. Left ankle
49. Tip of the left big toe
50. Tip of the second toe
51. Tip of the third toe
52. Tip of the fourth toe
53. Tip of the little toe
54. Left ankle
55. Knee
56. Hip
57. Lower abdomen
58. Navel
59. Center of the chest (heart)
60. Throat
61. Head

Once the journey is completed, feel the breath vibrating in the whole body, in the different points, from the top of your head to the ends of your feet, and from your feet to your head. Feel all the points vibrating simultaneously and radiating with the breath, as a backdrop that lights up in the silent space.

103. *Spinal breathing:*

*   As you exhale, mentally hear the sound *OM* and feel the energy flowing down from the top of your head to the tips of your toes; as you inhale with the sound *OM,* feel the flow of energy coming up from the tips of your toes to the top of your head. Observe your breath in this manner for a few moments.

*   Then, continue the same exercise—mentally hearing the sound *OM* and feeling the energy flowing down from the top of your head as you exhale and feeling the energy coming up as you inhale with the sound *OM*—from the top of your head to your ankles; then from the top of your head to your knees; then from the top of your head to the coccyx center; then from the top of your head to the sacral center; then from the top of your head to the lumbar center; then from the top of your head to the dorsal center; then from the top of your head to the cervical center; then from the top of your head to two points under your nostrils; from both the points under the nostrils to the cranial center, forming a "V" of vibration, sound, and light; then from the points under your nostrils to the top of your head.

*   Reverse the sequence—mentally hearing the sound *OM* and feeling the energy flowing down from the top of your head as you exhale and feeling the energy coming up as you inhale with the sound *OM*—going from the top of your head to the points under your nostrils, then from the top of your head to the cervical center; then from the top of your head to the dorsal center; then from

the top of your head to the lumbar center; then from the top of your head to the sacral center; then from the top of your head to the coccyx center; then from the top of your head to your knees; from the top of your head to your ankles; and from the top of your head down to the tips of your toes.

* This exercise can be simplified by staying only in the central axis, and allowing the breath to come and go from the coccyx center to the top of your head and from the top of your head to the coccyx center; or from the void between your feet to the void above your head.

* It can also be performed with another method of one's choosing, by repeating "I Am" instead of "*OM.*" As you inhale, feel the flow of energy rising in the spine, from your tailbone to the top of your head, and repeat "I" mentally. As you exhale, feel the flow of energy descending in the spine, from the top of your head to your tailbone, and repeat "Am" mentally, until the ebb and flow of vibrations envelop the whole body. Feel the awareness of being as you inhale, and the joy of being as you exhale, until the sensation, both feelings of being and the thought "I Am" merge in the tranquil, impersonal, still, and silent space, in which "All is One."

104. *Entering conscious sleep:*

* After the phase of spinal breathing, after any kind of exploration in the structures of the being, or simply at night when you go to sleep, it is important to become empty of all impressions, by allowing the attention to come back to its source.

* Start by letting go of the breath in the empty space of the head; breathe in this space for a few minutes, in order to become empty of all impressions associated with the waking state and the body. It is possible, without any particular effort, to listen to the vibration

of the sound *OM* radiating in this space, where all physical sensations are absorbed.

* Then, allow the attention to descend to the throat center, continuing the same process, as you become empty of the impressions associated with the dream state, allowing the gross vibrations, sensory impressions, emotions, thoughts, and images to dissolve in the empty space of the throat.

* After this, descend into the space of the heart, in order to become empty of all phenomena, memories, subtle vibrations, and especially of the sense of "me" or "I" performing a particular task, in a manner similar to the act of dying. Each exhaling breath must be experienced as the last one, in real terms, by completely disappearing in the empty pause, until a peaceful and thoughtless state, similar to that of deep sleep but with awareness, is revealed. In that moment, there is nobody left; there is no knowledge, no comment, neither desire nor aversion, and no "me," but only a restful state of total Awareness and undifferentiated bliss, in which all systems are regenerated. That is when the conscious perception of this state can reveal the very light that illuminates it, beyond the three states of waking, dreaming, and deep sleep. The witness of these states is neither awake, nor dreaming, nor sleeping; it is the space of Awareness in which all these states appear and disappear, like clouds in the sky. Awareness is present in all these different states, while remaining free of them and unaffected by them. It is the Being, without attributes, that cannot be seen, but that sees everything, the true nature of the Self, unborn, uncreated, omnipresent, that rests in itself by itself.

* At this "stageless stage," without duality, there is nothing to do or not do: the observer, the observed, and the observation are one, or they no longer exist. Regardless, its taste is beyond

words, concepts, descriptions, and thoughts. Simply being. If phenomena continue to arise, just remain as a welcoming space, without any intention other than simply being. Do not try to be this or that, or like this or like that; do not even try to be aware, awake, or I don't know what else, because all this only involves concepts that arise, and will continue to do so, in the dualistic mind. Being is not an object that can be obtained, that goes to sleep or wakes up. It simply is.

105. *Returning to sitting position:*

* While still lying down, after about ten minutes of simply being and simply welcoming the phenomena that appear and disappear, or in the morning after a night's sleep, when the first phenomenon arises from the depths of relaxation in pure silence, observe these phenomena for a few minutes, from the heart center. From there, stay in an available state, "remain open to the Opening," like the empty center of a wheel, the peaceful source that is naturally tranquil, from which everything emerges and unfolds.

* Notice the images, thoughts, and vibrations, the breath and sensations that come and go, without identifying with these phenomena, without trying to hold onto them or drive them away, but allow them to pass like clouds in the sky. Observe this for a few breaths.

* Then, with the same openness and the same profound peace, allow the attention to slide toward the throat center, welcoming the world of dreams and thoughts that continue to emerge, unfold, and disappear with each breath, in the peace of being-consciousness.

* Finally, the attention moves to the space of the head, from where the body is seen and intimately felt in its totality, once again noticing its shape, gravity, the five senses, where it is located in

the room, and so on. Feel that the body appears in the tranquil space of Awareness, and that, at the same time, this conscious space penetrates it completely. Feel the peace, the Awareness, and the joy of being infuse every cell, every thought, every breath, the whole universe and all beings.

* Then, with your eyes closed, stay as the witness of the body starting up again slowly, moving your hands and feet first, then turn to your left side for a few moments, before you gently come back to a stable and comfortable sitting position. During this phase, do not allow yourself to be carried away by the energy of the movement, but clearly perceive that the movement of the body appears in the tranquil and still space, as a witness of the action.

Meditation in a Sitting Position

106. Simply remain in a sitting position, and be present to what is. Do not try to do or to be anything in particular. Do not try to not do or to not be anything in particular.

* Simply be aware, effortlessly, of everything that arises in the silent space. This silent space is not an object of awareness: "I" am not aware of this space, but it is the space itself that is aware of everything that appears, including the so-called "I" who thinks he or she is meditating, which is just a thought among others. Observe this. There is meditation, but no one meditating. There is Awareness, but no one to be aware. Everything appears and disappears spontaneously, automatically, and effortlessly in this silent presence, which is still, uncreated, and unconditioned.

* Remain without the intention to do or to not do, and become aware that where there is no intention, there is no tension. Simply note that the sensation of the entire body arises naturally in Awareness, without any effort. The breath comes and goes naturally, effortlessly, and automatically. The same goes for the activities of the senses and thoughts: everything appears automatically; no one does or controls anything.

* Where does the ability to choose, decide, and reason come from? Notice the desire to move, but choose to not move. Who makes

this choice? Where does its cause come from? Observe, without thinking or reflecting. The "me" thought, "I am choosing" or "I am meditating" emerges in the space of Awareness. Observe this.

* Who can see this? Notice that all spontaneous answers (to this question) appear and disappear in the space of Awareness. It is possible to see a thought emerging and dissolving; the thought might steal all your attention and lead to a daydream, and this distraction may in turn be perceived, leading you to think and believe that "now, I am present, whereas a moment ago, I was absent." But who was present to this absence? If there is awareness of the so-called presence or absence, it means that awareness very much exists for one to be able to account for this. Observe this.

* Similarly, a thoughtless and blissful state is experienced, like during deep sleep. Suddenly, I realize that "I have come out of it." I then think, "Ah! That was so peaceful. Such peace! But I was unaware, I don't remember anything, I only know that it was peaceful." Who is saying this? If before there was only peaceful unawareness, and now there is awareness once again, there is definitely a witness who realizes this. Observe. Don't think. Stay calm. See how it is impossible to "stay calm." Take note of the fact that the one who wishes to remain calm cannot do so; and that the very thought or effort to do so disturbs the tranquility. See how this setback emerges in the tranquility itself. The peace is there, but there is nobody being peaceful. The being is naturally peaceful. And even before being peaceful, it simply is.

* All these words and all these comments are only an acknowledgment. During meditation, there is only silence aware of the silence. A silence in love with itself, which is eternal and unconditional. An "I Am" without form, name, attribute, or thought. You are That.

107. If, despite everything, meditation without object seems impossible at the moment, and if the restlessness is too significant and dominating, it is possible to lay the foundation in a conducive way and begin by effortlessly observing the coming and going of your natural breath.

* After a few minutes, observe the sensations in the body from the top of your head all the way down to your feet, and then from the ends of your feet to the top of your head, gradually, part by part, with utmost equanimity, and without reacting with desire or aversion to the sensations.

* When the sensations and vibrations in the entire body are clearly perceived, begin chanting out loud the sound *OM;* inhale deeply and chant the sound as you exhale, as slowly as possible. Be aware of the silent space from which the sound arises and into which it dissolves. Be aware of the pause with empty lungs at the end of every exhaling breath. After a while, continue to recite the sound mentally, more and more faintly, without effort; and then, simply listen to the sound with each breath, with the same awareness. Gradually, observe the silences lengthening naturally, and remain immersed in them for as long as possible, stopping the mental recitation.

* As soon as a thought arises, start the mental chanting again, until you plunge into silence once more. Repeat this as many times as is necessary, until only silence remains. In any case, and regardless of which method of meditation is chosen, chanting the sound *OM* may conclude a session, just the way it was started. *OM.*

108. *During subsequent activities (end):*
* Carry out your daily activities and allow them to take place naturally in the silent space, noticing your thoughts, words, actions, and your surroundings, from the moment you wake up until you fall asleep, every minute, day or night.

* If a phenomenon disturbs the inner tranquility, come back to tranquility by realizing that the phenomena itself emerges in this tranquility.

* If there is mental or emotional restlessness and the peaceful silence seems to be lost, recognize that the awareness of the restlessness is not restless, but the restlessness itself manifests in the conscious silence, the same way in which all movements of the body, the mind, and of nature in general appear and disappear in this impersonal and still presence.

* The witness of waking, sleeping, dreaming, and deep sleep is not awake, no more than it falls asleep, dreams, or is fast asleep. The witness welcomes all states that play out spontaneously. Life is a dynamic meditation, and every event, even the ones that are unfortunate, arises in this joy of being that can never leave us, because it is what we truly are. It is enough to simply recognize it.

PART II

EXPLORATION

Complementary Practices

Awareness of Tissues and Cellular Memory

Sophrology, also called "dynamic relaxation," uses breathing, relaxation, gentle movement, and visualization techniques to quiet the mind and ground one in the body. Caycedian Sophrology recommends beginning with a practice that focuses on each of the tissues of the body (skin, muscles, bones, and organs). This should be continued for a certain period of time (depending on one's sensitivity), in order to heighten awareness of the tissues.

Thus, in the technique presented here, each series of exercises related to the six centers (cranial, cervical, dorsal, lumbar, sacral, coccygeal) should be followed by a resting period, during which one should focus on a specific tissue, starting with the skin. As you inhale, become aware of your skin (in the corresponding zone or the whole body), and as you exhale, allow a feeling of pure happiness to emerge from the sensation. Repeat this process for as long as is necessary for the feeling of the skin and the joy emanating from this sensation to be well established. At the same time, remain open to all other phenomena that arise in the field of Awareness, without judgment or bias, always welcoming them, as if for the first time.

For a period of time ranging from several weeks to several months, the resting periods should only be used for this specific concentration.

Once the skin of the entire body has been made well aware of and profoundly felt, it is then possible to work in the same manner with the muscle tissue. When the muscle mass is felt as a mass of sensation and pure joy, it is possible to move on to the awareness of the bone tissue. Once the skeleton is properly felt, the concentration can be directed toward the organs. It is then useful to focus on the nervous system, by reinforcing the awareness of the brain and the spinal cord, in order to naturally open up to the perception of the energy circulating in the whole body, awakening a new quality of awareness and joy of being.

Little by little, the alert perception of the tissues will reinforce the awareness of the very life that animates them and integrates all their structures. And the perception of this blissful life will reinforce the presence of the silent welcoming space in which all phenomena arise, thus giving way to new therapeutic, existential, as well as spiritual horizons.

Caycedian Sophrology furthermore recommends that this process can be coupled with time dimensions. First, the present, due to the attention focused on the breath, and on the sensations and phenomena that appear, moment after moment.

Once the awareness of the body and the joy that goes with it are well established, the resting periods can be used for allowing a future situation to emerge; the subject can see himself or herself in this situation that is playing out very well, thanks to the awareness and joy of being felt in the present moment, when the situation is imagined. By repeating this exercise regularly, the mere thought of the situation will then be associated with physical relaxation and a joyful feeling, allowing one to tackle the situation in the best possible way when it finally arises. But the essential focus remains on the now, for the situation will arise in the now, just as the projection of the situation is appearing in the now. And this is why the importance does not lie in visualization or sweet daydreaming, but in body awareness and alertness in the present moment, in which everything appears.

The same goes for the memories that emerge in Awareness: past events are appearing in the now, and memories are also appearing in the now. Here and now, and no matter in what form it appears, the past only emerges as a thought. It only exists as thoughts, images, and memories. This fundamental realization can allow one to let go of repetitive and ruminative thoughts about difficult times, which prevent one from living peacefully in the present moment. The realization and discrimination that flow from this fundamental understanding will naturally allow one to make room for the present moment offering itself in the now, with less interference and discord relative to a past that no longer exists, and a future that does not yet exist.

In addition, the awareness of the tissues will also allow for the revealing of cellular (as well as molecular) memory and consciousness. Because the human cell carries in it the entire history of humankind, new phenomena can also emerge in consciousness, thus highlighting questions about transgenerational, prenatal, and postnatal issues, as well as questions about evolution. With the practice of Dynamic Meditation, the collective Awareness can also give rise to a new outlook on basic human values that emerge spontaneously from the depths of being, to be made flesh in the human body, extending the positive, productive, and balanced influence, from the family unit to all levels of society.

Hatha Yoga and Dynamic Meditation

This Dynamic Meditation, with its postures, breathing exercises, concentrations, and so on, constitutes an excellent introduction and add-on to the traditional practice of hatha yoga, and also involves the same physical, energetic, and spiritual approach used in mindfulness.

Even though this meditation can be practiced on its own, it can also be an integral part of a hatha yoga session. When done at the beginning of a session, it allows one to be deeply rooted in body awareness, thus awakening an attitude of presence to oneself, and an openness with which the other practices should be undertaken. The simple movements allow for the gradual warming up of the body's joints, thus enabling the practice, at a later stage, of specific poses that require more flexibility. Moreover, this meditation prepares the nervous system for the proper flow and conductivity of energy in the whole body, which is essential for the effective practice of yoga, and consistent with its traditional form, as described in the ancient scriptures.

The major poses of hatha yoga have already been described time and again in numerous books on the subject. It should also be stressed that these specific poses cannot be learned from a book; thus, it is important to take lessons from an able teacher, so as to study the postures properly, and receive correction or adjustment during practice; this can also help to avoid injuries and to commence a constructive practice, to which breathing exercises and concentration techniques, related to these poses, can be added. For this reason, in this book we will limit ourselves to a simple reminder of the most fundamental poses, using two traditional series that, taken together, constitute the perfect hatha yoga practice session.

As part of the Rishi Yoga Meditation, these series are naturally incorporated after or during the exercises involving the spine, when it feels like the right time to do so, but before the actual yoga nidra session (before exercise no. 100). That being said, it is important to take a few minutes to relax the body in a lying down position before beginning.

Sun Salutation (*Sūrya-namāskara*)

First and foremost, the famous Sun Salutation (*sūrya-namaskāra*) constitutes an excellent continuation of the Rishi Yoga Meditation. It is performed in the same way: slow movements with full awareness of the body, breath, and mind. Its daily practice is known to promote longevity, good health (by stimulating the endocrine system, making the joints, spine, and muscles more flexible, and more), strength, activation and flow of different energies, and so on. And this is why it constitutes an excellent preparation and a good warm-up (among other options and multiple variations involving the salutation), before practicing the actual poses.

The movements should be performed slowly; inhale one beat and exhale two beats, while chanting the sound *OM* mentally, on every exhaling breath. Allow the series to unfold in the still and silent space of Awareness.

1. Stand with your feet together in mountain pose (*tāḍāsana*), hands joined in the prayer gesture, and then inhale and exhale deeply.

2. Inhale as you raise your arms and push them slightly backward in the raised arms pose (*hasta-uttanāsana*).

3. Exhale as you bend forward in the hands to feet pose (*pada-hastāsana*).

4. Inhale and extend your right leg back in equestrian pose (*aśva-sanchalanāsana*).

5. Exhale and extend your left leg back in the four-limbed pose or plank pose (*caturaṅgāsana*), with your arms straight, and your back and legs aligned.

6. With empty lungs, place your body on the floor in the eight-limbed salutation pose (*aṣṭāṅgā-namaskāra*). Be aware of the contact of your feet, knees, hands, chest, and chin with the ground, with an attitude of reverence and surrender to the silent space.

7. Inhale and come to upward facing dog pose (*ūrdhva-mukha-śvānāsana*), with straight arms, relaxed shoulders, and your gaze turned upward.

8. Exhale, push down on your arms and straighten your legs in downward facing dog pose (*adho-mukha-śvānāsana*), keeping your heels on the ground.

9. Inhale and bring your right leg forward in equestrian pose (*aśva-sanchalanāsana*).

10. Now, exhale as you come to the hands to feet pose (*pada-hastāsana*).

11. Inhale as you raise your arms and push them slightly backward in the raised arms pose (*hasta-uttanāsana*).

12. And once again, exhale as you come to mountain pose (*tāḍāsana*), hands joined in the prayer gesture.

On the following inhaling breath, start the sequence again by raising your arms and pushing them slightly backward in the raised arms pose. Continue the exercise, and this time, extend your left leg back in equestrian pose for step 4 and left leg forward in step 9. Both these rounds constitute one series of salutation.

Sun Salutation (*Sūrya-namaskāra*)

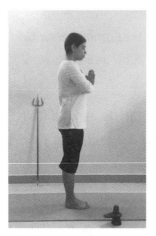 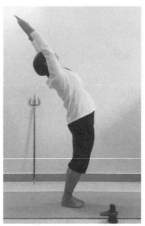 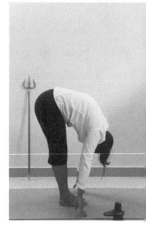

1. The mountain pose (*tāḍāsana*) 2. The raised arms pose (*hasta-uttanāsana*) 3. The hands to feet pose (*pada-hastāsana*)

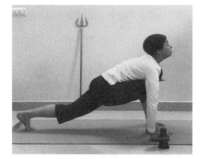 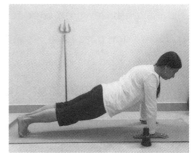

4. The equestrian pose (*aśva-sanchalanāsana*) 5. The four-limbed pose or plank pose (*caturaṅgāsana*)

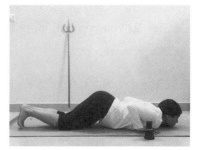

6. The eight-limbed salutation pose (*aṣṭāṅgā-namaskāra*)

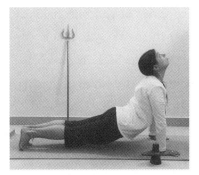

7. The upward facing dog pose
(*ūrdhva-mukha-śvānāsana*)

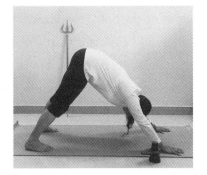

8. The downward facing dog
pose (*adho-mukha-śvānāsana*)

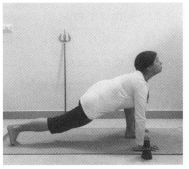

9. The equestrian pose
(*aśva-sanchalanāsana*)

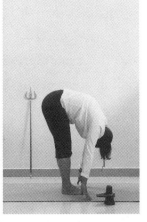

10. The hands to feet
pose (*pada-hastāsana*)

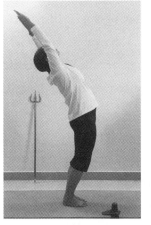

11. The raised arms pose
(*hasta-uttanāsana*)

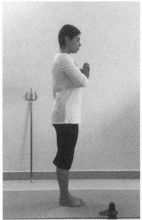

12. The mountain pose
(*tāḍāsana*)

Do six or twelve series of the Sun Salutation, always with full awareness and staying in the flow as much as possible, without any jerks. Then, lie down on your back in the corpse pose (*śavāsana*) and rest for a few moments, all the while observing your breath and the different sensations that come and go. Allow the breath to rise and fall in the spine. Feel the awareness of being as you inhale, and the joy of being as you exhale. Stay in this presence.

Rishikesh Series (*Rishikesh-kriya*)

With the same attitude to and awareness of the body, the breath, the energy flow, and the mind repeating the sound *OM,* it is then possible to continue the practice with a set of more specific poses. Do them in a coherent manner, so as to allow the energy to rise in your whole body through the spine, from the coccyx center all the way up to the void above your head, always going through each energy center located along the spine.

Of all the possible poses, there are twelve that stand out for their excellence. They also stand out for the power that only they have to bestow upon those who practice them: the stable tranquility so much sought after by yogis, in addition to balance, strength, joy, and good health. Known as the Rishikesh Series (*rishikesh-kriya*), and belonging to the Himalayan yoga lineage, these twelve postures are described below in an ascending order of the energy centers.

It should be noted, however, that it is possible to do this series in a slightly different order, by introducing alternative versions and additional poses. Even though one logically follows the play of energy, in reality that can only be understood with continuous practice and experience, and needs to be supervised by an able teacher. This holds particularly true when it comes to specific breathing exercises that go along with these different poses, in order to support the ascent and expansion of energy. But integrating these breathing exercises requires being very comfortable in the different postures. Therefore, in the basic version (version 1), it is important to breathe smoothly and deeply, inhaling one beat and exhaling two beats, unless indicated otherwise. So, here is a simple presentation that can be explored and adapted based on one's own experience.

Rishikesh Series (Rishikesh-kriya) Version 1

1. The triangle pose (*trikoṇāsana*):

* Stand with your legs spread apart, arms outstretched in the form of a cross and parallel to the floor; bend sideways (on one side, then the other), and place your hand on or next to your foot, which is turned outward; your other arm is raised and straight, pointing toward the void of the sky, and your arms are perpendicular to the ground; contract your anus, let your tongue turn backward, your gaze on your outstretched fingers positioned with the index fingertip touching the tip of your thumb.

* Allow the pose to settle in the silence, as you continue to simultaneously be aware of your breath, your big toes, anal region, abdominal region, thumbs, throat, eyes, and spine, and especially of the nostril in which the breath is flowing more freely, of the corresponding energy channel, and of the mind repeating the sound *OM*. The awareness is natural and effortless.

* With practice, the attention will first be focused on the ascent of the energy, boosted by the contraction of the anus; and then focused on the descent of the energy, captured by the hand pointing upward to the sky like an antenna, and with the arm acting as a channel for the energy flow. The energy is drawn in as you inhale, and it flows downward as you exhale. The perception of

this double movement reinforces the presence of the empty, still, and silent space in which the pose and the play of energy are taking place.

* Hold the pose for 3, 5, 7, or 10 breaths on each side; take time to feel the stimulation and neutralization of the lateral channels, before moving to the central path in the spine, with the practice of the following pose.

2. The hands to feet pose (*pada-hastāsana*):

* Begin in standing position, with your legs straight and feet together; inhale and raise your arms, pushing them slightly backward, then bend forward as you exhale; slide your hands under your feet and place your forehead on your knees; keep your back straight, your anus contracted, tongue rolled backward, and your gaze between the eyebrows. By combining the pose, the breath, and the sound, let the energy flow from the coccyx center to the cranial center.

* Hold the pose for at least two minutes.

3. The intense west stretch/seated forward bend (*paścimotānāsana*) or the ferocious pose (*ugrāsana*):

* Sit with your legs stretched out on the ground in front of you, and keep them straight like two sticks; grab your big toes with your thumbs, index, and middle fingers; tug on them gently in order to place your head between your knees, and stay still.

* Inhale as you draw the energy along the spine from the coccyx, sacral, and lumbar centers up to the cranial center; hold your breath for a few moments and allow the energy to spread everywhere in the still space; then exhale and let it come back all the way down.

* When you practice this pose, keep your anus contracted, tongue rolled back, and your gaze turned upward, so as to fully contrib-

ute to the rising of the energy. Stay open to the sensations, to the breath, and to the openness itself.

* Hold the pose for at least two minutes. Lie down on your back for a few moments, and enjoy the feeling by observing the breath come and go in the spine.

4. The cobra pose (*bhujaṅgāsana*):

* Lie down on your belly, place your hands on the floor near your shoulders, and simply raise your body (the part above the sexual organs) as much as possible, first without the help of your hands, and then by pushing with your arms; keep your shoulders down and relaxed, and raise your head like a cobra's hood. Make sure that your elbows are touching your sides. Keep the anus contracted, your tongue rolled back, and gaze turned upward.

* When you inhale, draw the sexual energy into the spine from the sacral center to the crown center, feeling it passing through the dorsal center; exhale slowly and let the energy come back down.

* Lastly, you could perhaps bring your heels to your buttocks, stick out your tongue and wriggle your pelvis, so as to rub and stimulate the sexual region, all the while continuing to draw in the energy. Allow the energy to rise like a snake, entering the spine and gushing into it.

* Hold the pose for at least two minutes.

5. The locust pose (*śalabhāsana*):

* Lie down on your belly with your chest on the floor, place both hands under your hips and raise both legs to a height of about eight inches above the ground; keep your gaze still and fixed on a point in front of you, your anus contracted, and tongue rolled back.

* By combining the pose, the breath, and the sound, let the energy

flow into the spine, from the lumbar center to the crown center, with the awareness of it going through the cervical center. Stay as a witness to the energy and the spreading heat that flows into the void.

* Hold the pose for at least two minutes.

6. The bow pose (*dhanurāsana*):

* With your legs spread out and your chest on the floor, hold your toes or ankles with your hands behind your back, and flex your body like a bow. Keep your anus contracted, tongue turned backward, and your gaze turned upward with your eyes open toward the empty space of the sky. Your arms remain relaxed, naturally and effortlessly straight as a result of the position of your legs. Your body is resting on your belly, from which the warm and vibrant energy rises and spreads to the empty and still space, through the whole body, by combining the pose, the gestures, the breath, and the sound. Allow the solar energy to spread freely in the sky.

* Hold the pose for at least two minutes.

7. The half lord of the fishes pose (*ardha-matsyendrāsana*):

* Sit with your back straight, and place your left ankle under your anus; bend your right leg so as to place your right foot on the outer side of your left knee, and turn your upper body and head to the right. Slide your left arm under your right knee and your right arm behind your back, and grip both hands together. Your gaze is between the eyebrows and is still, your anus contracted, and tongue rolled back.

* Once the pose is steady and comfortable, observe the breath rising and falling in the spine with the sound *OM*. Remain attentive to the play of the energy, the warmth, and the vibrations in your whole body and in the silent space that holds and embraces

everything. Gradually, the attention will focus on the stillness and on the attention itself, with the yogi remaining open to the openness, and the attention awakening to its own essence and to the profound peace, beyond all concepts about the internal and external.

✳ Hold the pose for at least two minutes on each side, being sure to notice the change in the breath passing through the nostrils, depending on whether the body is turned to the right or to the left.

8. The crow pose (*kakāsana*) or crane pose (*bakāsana*):
✳ Place your hands on the floor, place your knees on your arms, above your elbows and near your armpits, and lift your feet off the ground. Apply the root lock, tongue lock, and eyebrow center gazing gesture,* and observe your breath and the sound, as you let the vital energy gush through the central axis. Be aware of it passing through the heart and dorsal centers. Be like a bird, perched on a rock, observing, checking, and becoming aware of its surroundings and the boundless horizon, open wide before it.
✳ The peacock pose (*mayurāsana*)—more difficult to perform and in which the pressure of the elbows on the belly propels the energy in a powerful way all the way up to the crown—can be practiced in lieu of the crow or crane poses.
✳ Hold the pose for at least two minutes. Then rest for a few minutes on your back and enjoy the feeling, as you observe the breath coming and going in the spine.

---

*To apply the root lock, contract your anus, perineum, and genitals.

To apply the tongue lock, place your tongue above the soft palate and as far back as possible into the nasal cavity.

To apply the eyebrow center gazing gesture, roll both eyes upward and try to gaze at the eyebrow center.

9. The all-limbs pose or shoulder stand (*sarvaṅgāsana*):

* Lie down on your back and raise both legs slowly to the vertical position, supporting your torso with your hands and with your chin touching your chest. Inhale and become aware of the energy coming down from the sky, entering through your feet and flowing through the body to the cervical center. Exhale and enjoy the vibration spreading through the void in the throat. Be aware of the sound *OM* appearing and disappearing in the void, and surrender completely to this still and silent space.

* Hold the pose for at least two minutes.

* With a little practice, the straightened arms can be placed alongside your legs: this pose without support will reinforce dissolving in the still void. The pauses with empty lungs at the end of each exhaling breath become longer, in a natural way. The one who is practicing is completely set aside during these natural and spontaneous retentions of the breath. Then, there is nobody left to disturb the immense peace that fills up and embraces everything.

10. The plough pose (*halāsana*):

* Starting from the previous position, place your toes behind your head, as far as possible, with your legs straight; keep your arms on the floor with interlocked fingers. Keep sinking in to the void and allow the pauses after the exhaling breaths to become longer, aware of the body relaxing and dissolving in the silent space. This position has the ability to lessen the need for air generally required in normal breathing, and gives rise to a subtle breath, the resulting energy, a withdrawal of the senses, the effortless retention of the breath, the listening of the inner sound and of the silence.

* Hold the pose for at least two minutes, remaining as still as possible.

11. The fish pose (*mātsyāsana*):

* Come back to the all-limbs pose (*sarvaṅgāsana*) or start with the corpse pose (*śavāsana*), and take the lotus pose (*padmāsana*). Then use the support of your elbows and place the top of your head on the ground, all the while gripping each big toe with the respective hand. Apply the root lock, tongue lock, and eye lock. By combining the pose, the breath, and the sound, a sensation of floating sets in, thus allowing for total surrender and dissolving in an ocean of peace. Observe the current flowing from the lumbar center through the heart space and to the space above your head, in which your fixed and still gaze is lost. Stay attentive to the rivers of sensations, vibrations, and sounds finishing their journey in the vast ocean of emptiness.

* Hold the pose for at least two minutes. Rest for a few moments on your back.

12. The headstand (*śīrṣāsana*):

* Interlock your fingers and place your head on the ground against your hands; raise your legs slowly, until your body is straight like an "I": your belly is up and your palate is below. Allow your body to relax completely, with the breath and the sound. As you inhale, become aware of the energy from the sky that enters through your feet, and as you exhale with the sound *OM,* it flows into the body, going through the top of your head.

* Recognize the total stillness; your body is like a needle hanging in the void. Become aware of the profound regeneration of the different structures, and relax completely in the pose, which is performed without any effort. This royal pose is a total immersion in the void, the absorption of all forms of energy in their unique source.

* The scriptures say that the yogi who practices this for three hours daily, and who has dissolved in the immense void with

full Awareness, can overcome death, and is not destroyed by the destruction of the world. This is an image of course, but it says a lot about the power of this important pose.

* Hold the pose for as long as possible, and try to increase the duration by ten seconds every day.

Finish the practice session in the corpse pose (*śavāsana*) by lying down on your back for several minutes, and allow the different sensations, emotions, energies, thoughts, and images to dissolve in the conscious, deep, silent, and still tranquility. The session can end by resting in this manner, or you can continue with some breathing exercises as taught by a teacher, or with yoga nidra (exercises 100 to 105), and/or directly with meditation (exercise 106 or 107).

Rishikesh Series (Rishikesh-kriya) Variations

With practice, the yogi can include different variations in the series, change the order in which the poses are practiced, substitute some postures with others, add or remove certain poses, lengthen the duration for which the poses are held, add on breathing exercises or mantras, and so on, according to one's feeling, and/or depending on the spontaneity of the moment (different suggestions are presented in the illustrations that follow).

During the practice of the poses, it is important to observe the sensations with a lot of attention and equanimity, without reacting with desire or aversion, so as to not create any new memories, which will only further condition the reactions and ensuing suffering. This is why, by dealing with one's automatic resistances, the practice of postures allows for the acceleration of the process of the purification of these dormant impressions, and consequently, of the dissolving of conditionings, which is necessary for the total recognition of the joy and awareness of being.

While practicing these poses, and no matter which practice you choose, it is important to be alert without tension, to not focus on the resulting effects, to remain without expectations and with an attitude of availability and openness, in order to experience the omnipresent void. The yogi must fade away in the pose and be free of the belief that he or she is doing something, so as to allow another quality of intelligence, which is totally impersonal, to operate. From the pose itself, the yogi will always aim to open up to the conscious space in which the pose is unfolding, a witness to all the movements of the body and the mind. Then a time will come when, seeing that one cannot do this, one will dissolve completely in this realization and recognize that one is the silent space itself, free of the conditioned person. The joy of being will thus shine by itself, in itself, as the ultimate transcendence. There is yoga (union) and presence, but nobody to do or accomplish it: when the yogi disappears, Yoga is revealed. And only it remains; the eternal bliss that has never ceased to exist, and which will always be. *OM.*

Rishikesh Series (*Rishikesh-kriya*) Version I

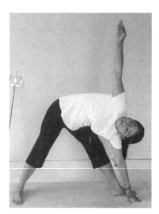

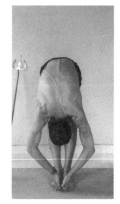

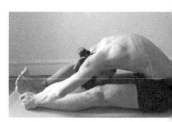

1. The triangle pose (*trikoṇāsana*)

2. The hands to feet pose (*pada-hastāsana*)

3. The intense west stretch/se forward bend (*paścimotānāsa* or the ferocious pose (*ugrāsaṇ*

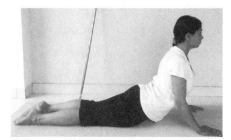

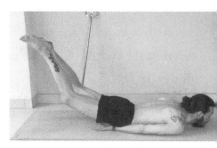

4. The cobra pose (*bhujaṅgāsana*)

5. The locust pose (*śalabhāsana*)

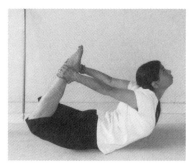

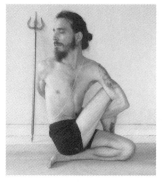

6. The bow pose (*dhanurāsana*)

7. The half lord of the fishes pose (*ardha-matsyendrāsana*)

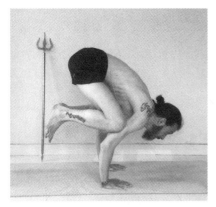

8. The crow pose (*kakāsana*) or crane pose (*bakāsana*)

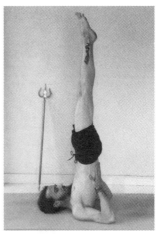

9. The all-limbs pose or shoulder stand (*sarvaṅgāsana*)

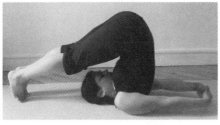

10. The plough pose (*halāsana*)

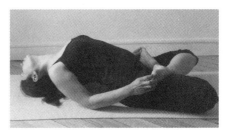

11. The fish pose (*mātsyāsana*)

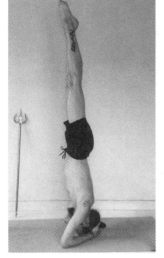

12. The headstand (*śīrṣāsana*)

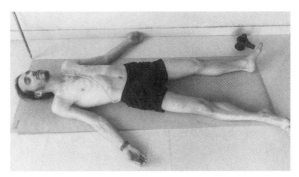

13. The corpse pose (*śavāsana*)

Rishikesh Series (*Rishikesh-kriya*) Version 2

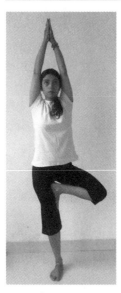

1. The tree pose
(*vṛkṣāsana*)

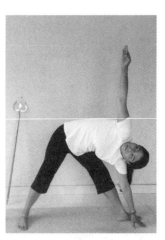

2. The triangle pose
(*trikoṇāsana*)

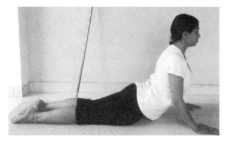

3. The cobra pose (*bhujaṅgāsana*)

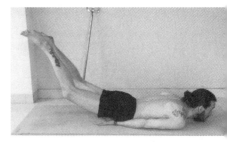

4. The locust pose (*śalabhāsana*)

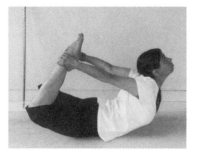

5. The bow pose (*dhanurāsana*)

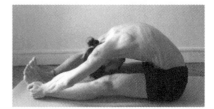

6. The intense west stretch/seated
forward bend (*paścimotānāsana*)
or the ferocious pose (*ugrāsana*)

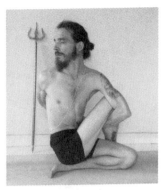

7. The half lord of
the fishes pose
(*ardha-matsyendrāsana*)

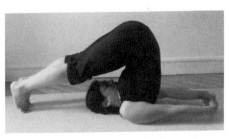

8. The plough pose (*halāsana*)

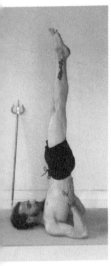

9. The all-
limbs pose or
shoulder stand
(*sarvaṅgāsana*)

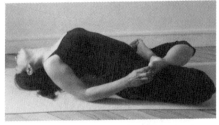

10. The fish pose (*mātsyāsana*)

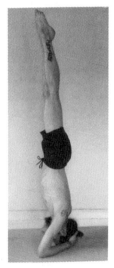

11. The headstand
(*śīrṣāsana*)

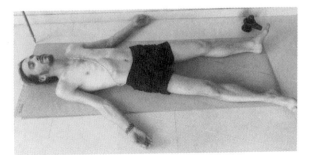

12. The corpse pose (*śavāsana*)

Rishikesh Series (*Rishikesh-kriya*) Version 3

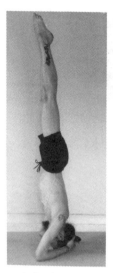

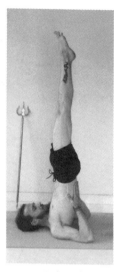

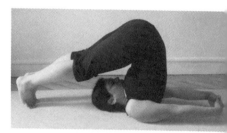

1. The headstand (*śīrṣāsana*)

2. The all-limbs pose or shoulder stand (*sarvaṅgāsana*)

3. The plough pose (*halāsana*)

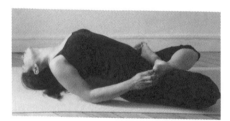

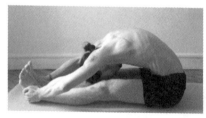

4. The fish pose (*mātsyāsana*)

5. The intense west stretch/seated forward bend (*paścimotānāsana*) or the ferocious pose (*ugrāsana*)

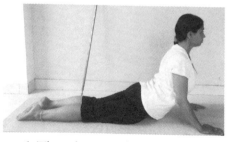

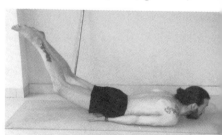

6. The cobra pose (*bhujaṅgāsana*)

7. The locust pose (*śalabhāsana*)

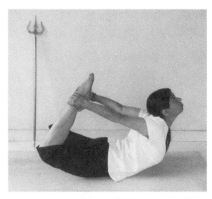

8. The bow pose (*dhanurāsana*)

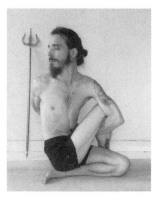

9. The half lord of
the fishes pose
(*ardha-matsyendrāsana*)

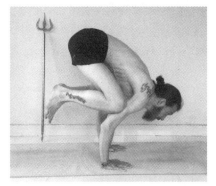

10. The crow pose (*kakāsana*) or
crane pose (*bakāsana*)

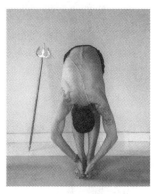

11. The hands to feet
pose (*pada-hastāsana*)

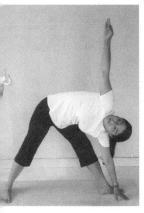

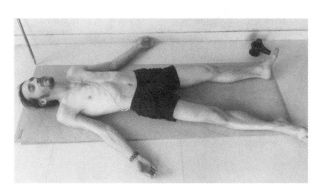

12. The triangle pose
(*trikoṇāsana*)

13. The corpse pose (*śavāsana*)

Rishikesh Series (*Rishikesh-kriya*) Version 4

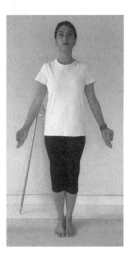
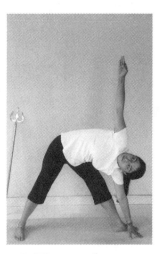

1. The mountain pose (*tāḍāsana*)

2. The triangle pose (*trikoṇāsana*)

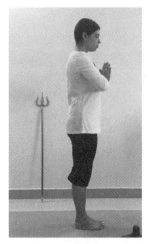
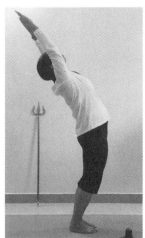
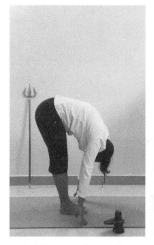

3. The mountain pose with hands in prayer mudra (*tāḍāsana*)

4. The raised arms pose (*hasta-uttanāsana*)

5. The hands to feet pose (*pada-hastāsana*)

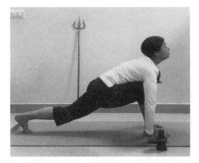

6. The equestrian pose
(*aśva-sanchalanāsana*)

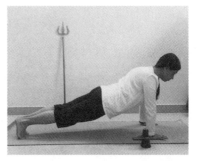

7. The four-limbed pose or plank
pose (*caturaṅgāsana*)

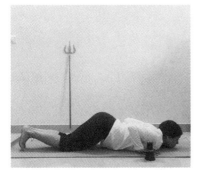

8. The eight-limbed salutation
pose (*aṣṭāṅgā-namaskāra*)

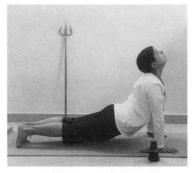

9. The upward facing dog pose
(*ūrdhva-mukha-śvānāsana*)

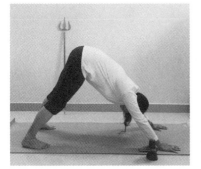

10. The downward facing dog
pose (*adho-mukha-śvānāsana*)

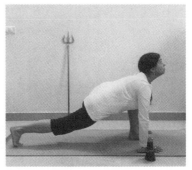

11. The equestrian pose
(*aśva-sanchalanāsana*)

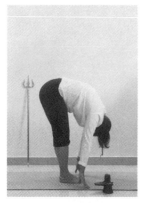 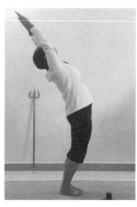 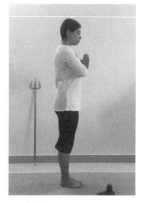

12. The hands to feet pose (*pada-hastāsana*)

13. The raised arms pose (*hasta-uttanāsana*)

14. The mountain pose (*tāḍāsana*)

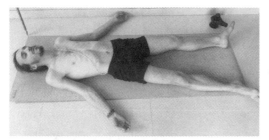

15. The corpse pose (*śavāsana*)

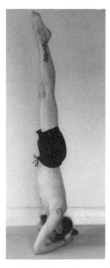 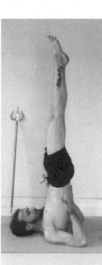 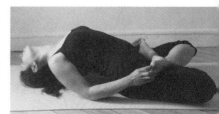

16. The headstand (*śīrṣāsana*)

17. The all-limbs pose or shoulder stand (*sarvaṅgāsana*)

18. The fish pose (*mātsyāsana*)

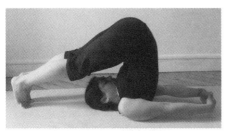

19. The plough pose (*halāsana*)

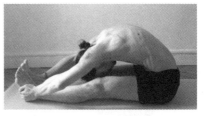

20. The intense west stretch/
seated forward bend
(*paścimotānāsana*)

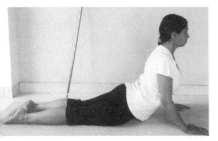

21. The cobra pose (*bhujaṅgāsana*)

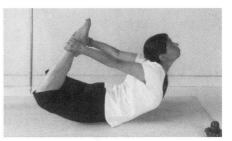

22. The crocodile pose (*makarāsana*)

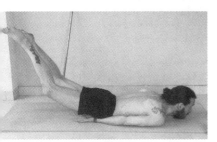

23. The locust pose (*śalabhāsana*)

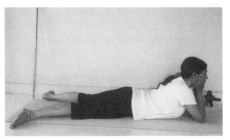

24. The bow pose (*dhanurāsana*)

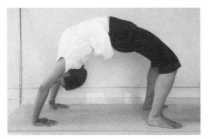

25. The wheel pose (*cakrāsana*)

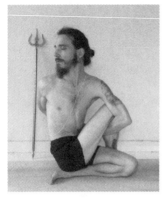

26. The half lord of the fishes
pose (*ardha-matsyendrāsana*)

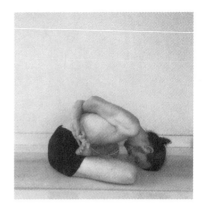

27. The gesture of yoga pose
(*yoga-mudrāsana*)

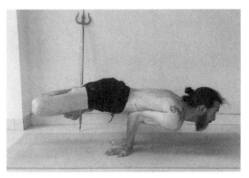

28. The peacock pose (*mayurāsana*)

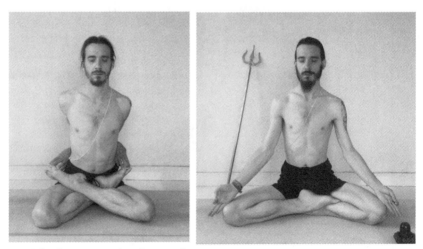

29. The lotus pose (*padmāsana*) 30. The meditation pose (*siddhāsana*)

Complete, Fast Session in Seven Steps

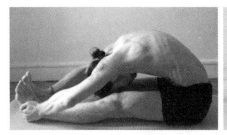

1. Flexion, forward folding: the intense west stretch/seated forward bend (*paścimotānāsana*)

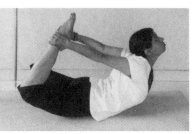

2. Extension, back-bending: the bow pose (*dhanurāsana*)

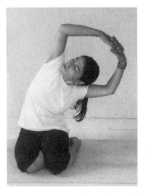

3. Lateral flexion, side-bending: the weighing-scale pose (*tolangulasana*)

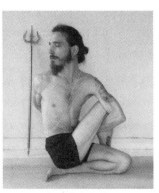

4. Rotation, twisting: the half lord of the fishes pose (*ardha-matsyendrāsana*)

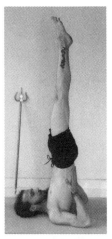

5. Inversion, going upside-down: the all-limbs pose or shoulder stand (*sarvaṅgāsana*)

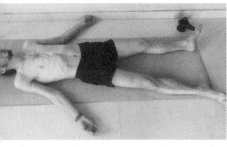

Relaxation: the corpse pose (*śavāsana*)

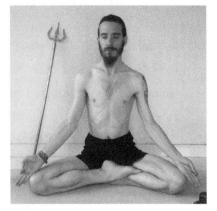

7. Meditation: the meditation pose (*siddhāsana*)

Notes on Yoga Nidra

Exercises 100 to 105, practiced in lying down position, constitute the basis of yoga nidra according to the Himalayan approach.* Although this practice can be done by itself, the body movements, hatha yoga poses, and breathing exercises constitute a wonderful preparation, which in turn effectively enhances the relaxation, sensitivity, withdrawal of the senses, concentration, meditation, and deep contemplation that yoga nidra gradually invites us to. The preparation allows one to have a better awareness of "that which is held on to" as much as of "the one who is holding on," so as to enable the final surrender that the yoga of sleep allows.

Yoga nidra goes far beyond the scope of deep relaxation: it allows for the recognition of the different structures of the being, and also of the different states of waking, dreaming, and deep sleep, thus shedding light on the conscious as well as the unconscious mind. When old conditioned memories rise to the surface, they are perceived and they dissolve, by the sheer force of awareness. Moreover, the alert perception of the phenomena and the different states essentially allows us to awaken to the very light that illuminates them, thus revealing that the awareness, the joy of being, and the recognition that pure being is our true nature, is not the result of some kind of practice or the

*For a complete, detailed, and practical presentation of this ancient science, read *Yoga Nidra Meditation: The Sleep of the Sages,* Inner Traditions International, 2017.

outcome of a particular phenomenon, but it is indeed the cause or the source of everything.

True happiness is not the consequence of an action, but the eternal reality that is prior to all manifestation. Pure Beingness or Awareness exists without the person, but the one who is practicing cannot exist without Beingness, which, by nature, is consciousness and bliss. The person manifests in pure Beingness, he or she is supported by Beingness, and will end up dissolving in Beingness itself, which always remains as it is, unchanging. One can then better appreciate Indian philosopher, guru, and poet Shri Aurobindo's words, when he states "Consciousness of being and Delight of being are the first parents. Also, they are the last transcendences." They are also the permanent support of all thoughts, words, and actions, the substratum present in the manifestation of all phenomena.

The repetition of the sound *OM,* for instance, clearly illustrates this: the sound emerges from and dissolves into the conscious silence, but this conscious silence is always present in the sensitive aspect of sound; it allows the sound to emerge, manifest, and then dissolve in its eternal embrace. The example with sound and silence might still seem a little dualistic, but this is not the case. In fact, language, which stems from thought, can only be expressed in dualistic terms, and it is thus unable to recognize pure non-duality, which is the essence of Beingness. To a certain extent, it is even possible to say that if there is awareness of sound and silence, or awareness of thoughts and of the absence of thoughts, it is only because there is awareness present to perceive all of this.

Therefore, "I Am" prior to all manifestation, and even prior to the emerging of the sensation, feeling, or thought that "I am," which is only a reflection of Beingness in the body-mind structure, like the sun reflecting in different puddles of water. This structure, believing that it is independent and separate due to identification, begins to seek and to practice, and to think it is doing something that will produce results, because of the sense of "me" and the ego. But when this identification ceases, things are then seen for what they truly are. The person, who is none other than a simple reflection, does not become free from anything, even though it may feel like that; but the Awareness, in a manner of speaking, is freed of the person. Then there is the realization of the boundless freedom of Awareness, which is always free by nature, with or without the person. Whatever is happening, whether one is standing, moving, or lying down like a corpse, only the unique taste of Bliss remains.

Therapeutic and Preventive Actions

The Rishi Yoga Meditation is a marvelous practice for promoting and maintaining global health and well-being of the body and the mind. The benefits gained through the practice of yoga, sophrology, and several other modern methods are clearly evident, and have already been written about extensively. So, in this book, we will only mention a few reminders and remarks relative to certain specific aspects of the approach suggested herein, as well as possible add-ons, in the event of the emergence of some general disorders.

By reinforcing awareness of the structures of the being, the suggested practices allow us to consciously work on harmonizing and rebalancing at different levels, thus providing an opportunity to be more self-reliant with respect to our physical and mental health, without having to fall back on external remedies, as far as possible, even though they are sometimes necessary. In the latter case, the remedies will be actively assisted by the practices, thus favoring external treatment. Without being an anatomy expert or a medical specialist, it is possible to acquire quick and simple resources for the setting-up of effective preventive measures, thus having a positive effect on common disorders, and alleviating potential suffering.

If mental agitation, stress, and anxiety are responsible for psychophysical disorders, a peaceful and conscious attitude, boosted by body awareness, breath control, and meditation, can prevent, control, treat, or eliminate them. This is naturally enhanced by a new outlook relative to nutrition, to sleep or waking patterns, recovery capacity, vital energy management, and so on. Yoga once again proves itself to be an art of living in its own right, embracing all aspects of our existence.

Rather than focusing solely on the symptom, which can lead to obsessions and ruminations, this global approach mainly seeks to strengthen all the positive aspects of the body and the mind. The inner peace and joy awakened by the movements, the poses, the breathing exercises, and the concentrations have a beneficial effect on the immune system, which itself optimizes its own work. During Dynamic Meditation, the conscious breaks can help this optimization, by always establishing a link between the physical, the energetic, and the mental, and with a proper intention. Given that each energy center is linked to specific vital organs, the amount of energy diffused in these organs can be combined, with an intention to improve their health and proper functioning. While inhaling, one mobilizes the energy in the center in question, for example, at the level of the dorsal center; while exhaling, one allows it to spread to the corresponding organs, such as the heart and lungs, focusing on the sensation of the body and on the feeling of happiness and well-being that awakens. As one continues to breathe, one allows the sensation and the feeling to infuse the organs, by trying, for example, to smile with all the cells of the organ in question, immersed in this deep relaxation.

This kind of preventive approach, when applied with full awareness, will have a positive effect on the body and the mind, as opposed to stress, negative emotions, and unconscious mental ruminations, which are the creators of physical as well as psychological disorders and malfunctions. To begin with, when one is dealing with a specific and localized symptom, the illness can be evoked mentally, along with its content and effects; the attention then moves to the physical region in question, and then to the closest energy center, both of which are generally related.

It is then possible to mobilize the energy from the center, by becoming fully aware of its vital force, and then diffuse it to the region that needs it, always with an intention of relieving, repairing, or healing. In situations where the energy is intensely felt in the whole body, especially in the central axis, it is possible to allow the vital force to flow directly in to the physical zone in question. By breathing in this region and sensing the vibrations, one allows it to simply purify itself and be energized, without thinking about the process, but instead allowing one's instinct to guide it.

Furthermore, several disorders arise due to a lack of energy, or due to some kind of obstruction or imbalance related to energy; the Rishi Yoga Meditation once again constitutes an excellent means of prevention, in so far as its movements work particularly on all the joints in the body. The joints are the junctions where the energy channels and meridians cross over, and every time this happens, they form small centers in which vital energy is stored, and then redistributed. Practitioners of traditional Indian medicine and of martial arts are very familiar with all these movements, which promote flexibility and a general awareness of the different centers, thus allowing one to maintain a harmonious flow of the vital energy in the whole body, and to anticipate potential obstructions.

While practicing the Dynamic Meditation, one can also massage these "hidden" (*marma*) points, in order to reinforce the effect of the movements. There are 108 principal points that cover the front and back of the body, the lower end of the body, as well as the arms, chest, and belly, and the back, head, and neck. Most of the points are quite large in size and easy to find because, in addition to the fact that many of them are located in the joints, they are often sensitive zones, like the temples, the base of the skull, or behind the knees. Touching and working on these points, through physical contact or mental concentration, will have an impact on the vital energy in the channels, thus affecting the physical, as well as energetic and mental structures.

The physical or energetic massage can be done by applying gentle pressure, with clockwise movements to stimulate the point, and counterclockwise movements to remove blocked energy. The focus of the attention, as practiced in certain concentrations, is synchronized with the vital breath, the physical sensation, and the intention. It is thus possible to stimulate, appease, protect, diffuse, and energize, according to the needs of the moment. For example, a painful knee can be massaged physically. This action can also be combined with inner work: while inhaling, mobilize the vital energy in the knee, and while exhaling, allow the pain to fade away by becoming aware of the pleasant irradiation of the energy in the bone structure, the tendons, and the flesh, and in the space all around. This is just another example to illustrate the basic principle, because, once again, what is essential is to allow our instinct to adapt to the needs of the moment.

The recognition of the profound silence and of the joyous feeling of energy allows us to open up to a more intuitive and impersonal dimension, which is non-codified, obeying the inherent intelligence of Awareness itself, and opening up to that which is beyond technique and basic knowledge. The stopping of the mind allows for a new outlook on all internal and external phenomena, which is free of the conditioned judgments that restrict us to common, fixed, and simplistic patterns, fueled by biases.

This stopping unleashes creativity, intuition, adaptability, integration, and all possibilities, beyond pre-established knowledge, and in that respect, it better serves to solve a problem than regular mental reactions.

Once we have learned the key points and principles, common sense, attention, experience, and intuition become the best guides. The links between the different structures and means of action are revealed naturally, beyond simple knowledge, in the inner tranquility and correct observation of the centers. Letting go, especially of the desire to control everything, unleashes an impersonal intelligence that abides in each one of us, which flows through us and molds us, in the empty space of Awareness where all tensions are released, naturally and effortlessly.

A more conscious attitude allows one to adapt more intuitively to the context and to the seasons, to assimilate the techniques and the way to practice, and to develop natural and spontaneous therapeutic responses within oneself, based on an actual practice of prevention. Moreover, every practice, no matter how simple it may be, can be the stepping-stone to ever-blissful Awareness. Laughter, for instance, or singing, or any other kind of enjoyment, acts as a marvelous medicine for the body and the mind, but these moments are also wonderful opportunities to recognize the Awareness prior to them. For the essence is beyond sickness and health, in the Beingness that never changes, and which is blissful by nature, that yoga encourages us to recognize, in order to become one with that which is never ill, with that reality untouched by sickness, old age, and death.

Suffering from a disease can be the opportunity to realize the Self, which is naturally free of all suffering. Meditation indeed leads to the recognition that the one who witnesses the suffering does not suffer, and that the witness of the disease is not sick. Meditation allows for the revealing of the unchanging reality, beyond sickness and health, and beyond constantly changing phenomena. Indeed, therein lies the aim of yoga. Therefore, no matter what happens, we can remain peaceful, internally unaffected and free of everything, whether our body is healthy or not. It is an awakening to the everlasting joy that surpasses external mechanisms conditioned by nature. And therein lies the most beautiful gift that yoga has given us: the discovery of fundamental and blissful Oneness, in all circumstances.

Investigating the Structures
of the Being

At this stage of the practice, it is possible to explore the different structures of the being one by one, in a precise and keen manner, by focusing on one specific aspect or another, in a gradual and systematic way, especially during the conscious resting periods after each series of movements, or after the spinal breathing exercise (practiced seated or lying down).

Focusing on the Six Energy Centers

It is possible to come up through the energy centers, always starting at the base center, and moving from the gross centers toward the subtler ones, stopping at each center in order to concentrate on a particular phenomenon, and then going back to the unique source of all manifestation. With this aim in mind, the inquiry will first focus on the states of matter, and then on the states of awareness and the structures of the being associated with each state, always seeking to examine and understand the essential nature of the one who claims to carry out this inquiry.

According to this logic, which belongs to different points of view of Indian philosophy and traditional yoga, the base energy center, located at the level of the coccyx and the anus, can be the starting point for concentrating on the earth element or the solid state. In order to do this, one can become aware of one's skin, muscles, bones, organs, and one's entire physical structure, also allowing this awareness to spread to the ground on which the body is resting, and to all internal and external solid material. The concentration is more effective when it is synchronized with the breath: when you inhale, let the sensation of the earth element emerge, and when you exhale, allow the feeling that this unique sensation brings to emerge, which, in this case, corresponds to a sense of solidity, stillness, and utmost tranquility. There is nothing to imagine or create: everything is already here and it is only a matter of recognizing it.

The clear perception of solidity will naturally reveal the awareness of the water element, which is subtler, and whose gravity center is located, in a matter of speaking, in the sacral center in the pubis region. The water element corresponds to the liquid state: not to the liquids in the body, per se, which belong to the earth, but to the rivers of energy and to the currents of vibration that inhabit and flow through the physical body. The concentration, synchronized with full awareness of the breath will, as noted above, gradually reinforce the sensation of the currents of vibration that go beyond the limits of the skin, and allow a feeling of fluidity, reassurance, well-being, and tremendous vitality to emerge.

By maintaining this concentration, the perception of the water element will give rise to awareness of the fire element and the igneous state: the attention will shift to the lumbar center, in the solar plexus region, and the sensation will continue to spread, with a powerful feeling of the vibrations accompanied by heat and light, which will begin to burn the sense of "me" and the feeling of doership. If alertness and equanimity are maintained, the process will then begin to awaken a more and more impersonal feeling, wiping out ordinary limits of perception and effort.

The energy focus will naturally move upward to the dorsal center, in the heart region, awakening an awareness of the air element and the gaseous state, corresponding to a sensation of all-embracing, limitless, and impersonal energy that, in turn, awakens a feeling of pure joy, freedom, and ever-expanding awareness, as though it were possible to touch the whole universe.

The awareness of this very subtle phenomenon, related to the air element, can then awaken one to the consciousness of the space in which the very feeling of expansion emerges, thus revealing the unique sense of profound stillness that contains everything. Even though the gravity center of the space element is located in the cervical center, in the throat region, it is possible that, at this stage of the practice, any geographical or physical reference dissolves completely, along with the sense of "me" as being something specific or being in a particular state.

If this is not the case, and if the feeling of being a person concentrating on something persists, it is then possible to do the following: while inhaling, become aware of the formless and limitless silent space, and while exhaling, surrender completely and allow all phenomena related to sensations, vibrations, feelings, thoughts, images, visions, and so on, to dissolve completely, until only total stillness remains, without any thoughts.

Upon reaching this point, where there is neither anything left to do nor anyone to do it, it may become possible to recognize that the essential nature of Awareness is neither earth, nor water, nor fire, nor air, nor space, nor any experience or state, but the unchanging witness of them all. In this recognition prior to all thoughts, even the notion of being the witness, the awareness, or anything else, is absent. Any kind of knowledge has disappeared, but Awareness remains, aware of itself, in a manner of speaking. But even this is still a concept belonging to the mind, for where there is no mind, there is nothing left to say. Only silence remains.

This kind of practice is bound to raise the most fundamental questions: who is practicing? Who am I? The problem always lies in taking oneself to be the doer of an action, in believing that one is doing something, and consequently, that one is a person who is failing or succeeding. The inquiry can now focus on the nature of this "I" or "me" who believes that he or she is someone doing something in particular, who consistently identifies with experiences, situations, names, and forms. Who is this "I" or "me"? And where is it located? Even though this sense of "me" or this feeling of "I" is only a pale reflection of pure Awareness or joy, it can be a useful guide for going back to that unborn and eternal source, which is always present, regardless of the situation and the experience.

Focusing on the Sheaths

In the same manner as with the concentration on the elements, it is also possible to explore the different layers or sheaths before letting go of them. In keeping with Indian philosophy, the attention will first focus on the grossest structure and gradually lead to the recognition of the most subtle structures. It is as if one were peeling an onion, until the empty center reveals itself. The empty center can also be seen as the center of a wheel, without which not only would the wheel be unable to turn, but it simply would not exist. Regardless of the phenomenon being observed, it is necessary to first concentrate on it, by focusing one's attention and thought exclusively on that specific area: awareness while inhaling and penetration while exhaling. Slowly, the attention, by focusing exclusively on one point, moves beyond ordinary mental concentration, and becomes meditation. Finally, when the attention is directly connected with that which has no form, through the object up to its formless essence, there is contemplation; a merging takes place, and subject-object duality dissolves, making room for a state of Oneness and spontaneous recognition.

In practice, this is a step-by-step process, from the gross to the subtle, by undoing one blockage after another, and by letting go, layer after layer, until reality is revealed on its own. And it is the combination of deep relaxation and very fine attention that allows this opening to the original Vision and to the conscious space of the all-embracing and all-pervasive relation, free of the observing and the observed.

The exploration thus starts at the physical body composed of food. Step by step, one concentrates on the presence of one's body, its location, form, gravity, weight, and mass, and also on one's skin, muscles, bones, organs, glands, nerves, blood, and fluids, as well as on the sense organs and organs of action, all composed of solid foods and liquids that have been absorbed. One senses the solid, the liquid, the igneous (heat), and the gaseous (air) matter, as well as the space, inside and outside, and all around one's body. Once one becomes aware of the presence of this seemingly solid matter, it is reinforced by becoming aware of the sheath as one inhales, and by letting the attention penetrate it as one exhales, all the while remaining conscious of the joy that emerges from this sensation, until the essence is revealed in deep contemplation.

The gravity center is located at the level of the base energy center, associated with the earth element, with the solid state, with the waking state, and the sense of a physical "me." This awareness is effortless: if I am aware of the body, it means that I am not the body, and that it simply manifests in the awareness, along with transformations like old age and disease. The body changes, but the awareness of these changes does not change.

The exploration continues with the subtle body corresponding to the energetic structure, the link between the body and the mind, which is of particular interest to us in yoga, because it offers a variety of avenues to be explored, especially in the practice of yoga nidra. Based on various methods, one concentrates on the different elements of this structure composed of the food of vital air and energy. These elements are primarily the vital breaths (of respiration, excretion, digestion, belching, and so on), the energy channels, and the energy centers. Once one becomes aware of the presence of this seemingly liquid or vibratory structure, it is reinforced by becoming aware of the four phases of subtle respiration, of this sheath of vibrations that enters and encompasses the physical body as one inhales, and by letting the attention penetrate it as one exhales, all the while remaining conscious of the joy that emerges from this sensation, until the essence is revealed in deep contemplation.

The gravity center is located at the level of the sacral region, in the sexual region, associated with the water element, with the liquid state, and with the sense of a vital "me." However, if I am aware of these energy currents (in my legs, arms, torso, neck, head, spine, and so on), of this vital structure linked with the breath, it means that I am, yet again, other than all of this. It is not "me" who is breathing; the breathing and vibrating is happening on its own, automatically and effortlessly.

The exploration of the subtle body continues with the mental and emotional structure. One concentrates on automatic thoughts (doubts, questions, answers, and so on) and emotions (desires, aversions, and fears), made up of sensory impressions, in the navel and mental space. The mind feels and receives external stimuli through the five senses, which creates a continuous flow of mechanical thoughts. It is merely about remaining as the observer of the process. The gravity center is located at the level of the lumbar energy center, in the abdominal region, associated with the fire element, with the igneous state, and with the sense of thinking and an emotional "me." Here, it is important to have equanimity, to remain very alert, and to allow the thinking and perceiving "me," which is only the result of identification and of the interaction between the senses, the breath, and the mind, to burn in the fire of attention. If I am aware of the five senses, of emotions, of pleasure and suffering, and of the mental phenomena that appear and disappear on their own, without any effort, it means that I am, yet again, other than all of this. There is nothing to control, manipulate, or change. Everything happens automatically.

The exploration of the subtle body continues with the intellectual structure. You observe reflective thinking, intuition, and the sense of an individual "me" (individuation or the process of individuating), composed of instant impressions and memory. For example, you can focus on the spinal breathing and count each inhale and exhale, starting from zero, as you continue to notice other thought phenomena rising, disturbing the counting or superimposing themselves on it, without ever stopping it. Observe the breaks in the counting as well, and how one comes back to it.

Make the decision to stop counting; and then decide to start counting again. Observe and recognize the phenomenon that counts, decides to stop and start again, which detects and determines the action. Who is counting? Who decides to stop or continue? With this feeling, begin a countdown with synchronized respiration, from twelve to zero, counting one inhalation plus one exhalation as one; allow the breath to lead the "me" to the heart of yourself, to the "person" you believe that you are, who takes himself or herself to be the doer of this action. The presence of this intellectual structure is reinforced by mentally repeating "I" as you inhale, and "Am" as you exhale. Observe the thought "I Am" repeating, emerging and disappearing in the space of Awareness; it is also possible to ask yourself when this sense of "me" appeared for the first time.

Welcome the phenomena and allow memories linked with choice-making or decision-making moments. Be aware of the cause and the doer of these actions. Be aware of the creation of the intellect (made up of thoughts and conditioned desires) that thinks, analyzes, has great ideas, and decides which response must be given to different stimuli. Observe. Contemplate the flow of thoughts. Who is contemplating? Who is deciding? Who is this "me" that believes it is contemplating, doing something, and performing a task? Who claims authorship of every action, perception, feeling, or thought? Be aware of the nature of this authorship: its name, form, memories of past experiences, hopes about the future, and habits. Allow an image of this "me" to emerge. Who am I? To whom do these responses and thoughts appear? Who is afraid of losing what you have (like your house, job, family, and life)? Who refuses to serve others graciously? Who is afraid of disappearing or dying? Who desires or wants to live? Who believes that he or she is the body and these thoughts? Notice that all responses are only mental events, only thoughts.

The gravity center is located in the energy center of the heart, associated with the air element, the gaseous state, and the thinking sense of "me" in general, the "I-me" sense. If I ask myself, "Who am I?" the answer is inevitably "me," or perhaps other concepts such as "awareness," "the witness," "light," "the Self," "space," and so on. Conscious of these manifestations, I am none of them. I am not anything perceptible, visible, expressible, or conceivable. Even this so-called "I" that claims to be neither this nor that remains elusive, as if it does not exist. The reality that observes is prior to the manifestation of any thought or claim, be it verbal, mental, or implied, forming in the mind. This reality is free of the thought of being someone who exists, does, or observes something. This conditioned thinking belongs to the intellect, but this reality is not the intellect, which is a mere reflection of the former.

The exploration continues with the causal body or the structure of bliss. Observe the unawareness similar to that of deep sleep, made up of dormant and unmanifested impressions. In order to do this, simply be a spectator to the flow of thoughts, emotions, images, and impressions that the mind receives, and feel the space in which these phenomena arise, how they reflect in the mind, and the space in which they dissolve. Simply notice that everything that emerges in the unawareness defines and conditions the mechanical nature of the mind, the intellect, the sense of "me," words, and actions. Observe how habits and unconscious memories are colored by reactions of desire and aversion, and how they influence the mind (and actions) in the absence of an active intellect that should be making all the decisions.

Observe how the unawareness emerges in consciousness, how it manifests. The presence of this seemingly empty matter, which is spatial, is reinforced by remaining in the simple observation of every phenomenon that appears and disappears, all the while remaining aware of the profound bliss that emerges from this sensation, until the essence is revealed in deep contemplation. The gravity center is located in the throat energy center, associated with the space element and the state of emptiness. The sense of "me" does not exist here, hence the absence of suffering and duality, and the presence of a feeling of joy and immense peace, as in deep sleep. But upon returning to the waking state or thinking state, the sense of "me" claims the experience, thinking, "I experienced this or that." This break, this unawareness or temporary absence, rekindles the thinking, perceiving, and operating "me." One can thus call it the "causal me." In fact, concentration is impossible at this stage, because there is nobody left to concentrate or even to give the command to do so. It is a kind of spontaneous recognizing.

In case thoughts persist, the only thing to do is to keep

observing or repeating a sound like *OM,* until the intellect that repeats it dissolves in this undifferentiated mass of impersonal awareness. Allow the clouds of phenomena to pass through and be absorbed in this blissful space, without thought or feeling. Allow accumulated memories to dissolve, and conditionings to come undone.

The Himalayan tradition considers this paradoxical state, which combines the peace of deep sleep with the alertness of the waking state, empty of thoughts, to be the stage where yoga nidra truly commences, not as a technique, but as a state. However, if there is awareness of an absence or of a state of unawareness, it means that some reality is still present to observe it, in silence. The witness of the one who is asleep is not asleep. The experience has the taste of oblivion, but the experience and the taste themselves are just ephemeral manifestations. The bliss that is experienced in this state is, once again, merely a reflection of a greater Bliss. The reality is, once again, beyond remembering and forgetting.

If a particular state is experienced, even if it is a state of absence, of being or non-being, it means that Awareness is there, present in the background of the experience, to experience it. This is how, by letting go of this very subtle object of experience, the Awareness can awaken to its own essence, without name or form. To whom does this bliss or this absence appear? Is it temporary or permanent? Who is aware of the states of waking, dreaming, and deep sleep? Actually, there is nobody left to even ask the question. Here, there is only Beingness and Awareness, love, bliss, and eternity, pure Presence prior to all manifestation and phenomena. These are, yet again, merely words; but it has become clear that, no matter what one says or thinks about it, the awareness of that which changes does not change. The awareness of the presence and absence cannot be objectified, measured, qualified, or spoken about. It is neither a sensation, nor an emotion, nor a feeling, nor an idea, nor an experience, nor a state, nor a phenomenon. And, because it is not something happening to someone, it is not even a revelation. If there is nobody left to observe, then nobody can claim to be the witness. It simply is.

PART III
REFLECTION
Philosophical Perspectives

Different Approaches to Awareness

The word *reflection,* from the Latin word *reflectere* meaning "to turn back," indeed refers to the act of reflecting or thinking, of stopping to consider something and examine it in detail; but it also designates the phenomena through which waves, vibrations, or light reflect off a surface. What is being described here is not intended to make us think about something in order to resolve an issue intellectually, but rather to draw our attention beyond thoughts and words, which are only fragile and changing reflections of a vaster reality, of an omnipresent and silent surface on which the sensitive aspect of thoughts, words, and the world is reflected. In the silence of the being, this uniting essence is revealed, allowing us to understand that nothing is separate from that which is already everywhere and that everything points to it. Each word, like a wave, rises and falls within it; and the words are only an invitation for the alert reader to dive into the bottomless and formless ocean of the joy of being. Although it may seem like a path has been traced, there is, in fact, nothing to do and nowhere to go. For the center of Bliss, of presence without boundaries, is already everywhere, here and now.

Yoga: Phenomenology and Full Awareness

Patañjali's Yoga Sūtras, written over two thousand years ago, summarize the teaching of one of the six important points of view of Indian philosophy. His 195 yoga aphorisms (*yoga-sūtra*) explore the body-mind structure within us by inviting us to recognize, through self-observation, the blissful nature of Awareness that illuminates every moment of our daily life. They constitute a meaningful synopsis of "mindfulness," which is concise, brief, easy to remember, and useful to recall.

The practice of yoga is accessible to all, irrespective of one's religion, culture, gender, or age; it allows one to be free of the conditioned behavior of the body and the mind, and allows one to enjoy a life in which everything is joy and acceptance of what is. The technique and process of purification explained by Patañjali have many points in common with those given by the Buddha in his text about establishing attention (*satipaṭṭhāna-sūtra*) and in *vipassanā* meditation. In the same manner, implementing these teachings can free one from suffering. Therefore, they "help to reduce stress and depression," as it is customary to say nowadays. But yoga is neither a self-help method, nor a gentle exercise routine for relaxing, nor a violent effort that wears down the body, and even less a way to enhance the appearance and well-being of the petty individual; far from it. The freedom that Patañjali evokes is not *for* the person, but *of* the person; the "I-me" should give way to "I Am." Understanding this difference is a discovery in itself.

Patañjali discusses the discipline of yoga as it is described in the revealed texts of the *rishis,* the visionary sages of ancient India. Although the Yoga Sūtras represent a fundamental text about yoga from a philosophical point of view, they belong to a more ancient lineage, which is the direct oral teaching passed on continuously from master to disciple.

The text composed of 195 aphorisms is divided into four chapters. An expert in the human psyche, Patañjali begins by telling us what the aim is in the first chapter (*samādhi-pāda*), because no one studies anything without knowing why. It is no coincidence that Heidegger said (on a relative note) that it is the future I project that gives meaning to my present: I must have a glimpse of where I am headed to want to go there. The first chapter, with 51 *sūtra,* mainly talks about contemplation (*samādhi-pāda*), which is the aim of yoga and which is yoga itself. In it Patanjali gives a clear definition of yoga, describes the observation of five types of thought, the principles of the practice and of non-attachment, the stages of concentration, efforts, commitments, obstacles, and solutions that stabilize the mind.

The second chapter (*sādhana-pāda*) gives a step-by-step explanation of the practice. The third chapter (*vibhūti-pāda*) is about the effects of the practice; and the fourth (*kaivalya-pāda*), like the Buddha's sermon in Sarnath, sings praises of the liberation from suffering relative to the phenomenal world.

The whole subject is beautifully summed up by the first four aphorisms, with a conviction that is rare. The remaining aphorisms, which can be subjectively divided into eighteen sections, are an explanation of the first four, and nonetheless very precious in guiding one's practice.

अथ योगानुशासनम्॥ १ ॥
Atha yogānuśāsanam||1||

1. And now (*atha*) begins the teaching (ānuśāsanam) of yoga (*yoga*).

The practice begins immediately, here and now (*atha*). I cannot practice yesterday or tomorrow; it is impossible. Tomorrow only exists in the now. So, if I spend my time putting off until tomorrow what I can do today, it is certain that I will never do it, because tomorrow does not exist. There is only now. When Husserl evokes the "living present," he is talking about that which is taking place, namely phenomena. In this context, the present is inextricably tied to the conception of the past and the future, to the phenomena of "retention" (perception retained in consciousness) and "protention" (anticipation of the next moment). Usually, when I say that I am "enjoying the present moment," I am referring to that which is present here, to that which is taking place. But, the "here and now," so dear to the Zen tradition as well as to yoga, refers less to that which is taking place than to the space of Awareness in which everything is happening, and in which all phenomena appear and disappear. This includes what we refer to as the past, the present, and the future. And this is indeed where everything begins, in this Presence to the present; and it is also where everything ends, from where it all emerges and where it all dissolves.

Receiving this teaching and aspiring to more awareness calls for being more available "now" (*atha*), which is the first word of the text. There is nothing more important than knowing myself, than going beyond my own basic notion of myself. The word *atha* marks the beginning of the practice and implies that one must prepare for it, through life experiences, and that one must be mature, in a manner of speaking, and sufficiently eager to release oneself from suffering, eager to know the awareness and boundless joy that are consubstantial to oneself. Before, I used to live in darkness; now, I am living in light. When the student is ready, the teacher will appear.

And so, here is the teaching that begins now, opening up a sacred and auspicious space here, which I must connect with, unite with (*yoga*), and be totally committed to, so as to be the incarnation of this traditional teaching (*śāsanam*), belonging to a continued lineage (*anu*), with a systematic learning method to be implemented, which is described in this book. This method is more about listening well than making any kind of effort, more about letting go than wanting to control, and more about passive observation than wanting to do something. Yoga is simultaneously a teaching and a quality of being. It is more a question of observing and understanding the states of mind for the purpose of transcending them, as if the perception of a noisy mind can not only reinforce the understanding of this kind of process, but also the awareness of Awareness itself, which is always silent and empty by nature.

According to the sage Vyasa's first comments on Patañjali's aphorisms, the mind, in its pathological or lucid aspect, can present five different types of behavior (*vṛtti,* pronounced as *vritti*):

1. The mind can be agitated (*kṣipta*), constantly evolving, propelled (*kṣip*), without control, and essentially driven by the energy of movement (*rajas*).

2. The mind can be confused, astonished, lost (*mūḍha*), lethargic, asleep, drowsy, depressed, and essentially driven by the energy of inertia (*tamas*).

3. The mind can also be scattered or distracted (*vikṣipta*) and essentially driven by a mix of movement and inertia (*rajas-tamas*), like when one forgets to focus on one's breath during meditation; it just comes and goes, like a monkey jumping from one tree branch to another, from desire to aversion, to suffering.

4. Concentrating on a single point (*ekāgra*), as Patañjali recommends in the practice of yoga (from the word *yuj,* meaning "to harness or to integrate"), or of reduction (from the Latin word *reductio,* which means "to bring back"), reduces stress and suffering. This quality of concentration is supported by a stable mind (*sattva*).

5. *Ekāgra* can give way to a suspended or suppressed (*nirodha*) mind.

The first three types of mental behavior prevent one from recognizing Awareness (*samādhi*); the fourth makes it available, and the fifth opens up to this spontaneous realization in which thought fades out and gives way to pure Presence, which by nature is free of the qualities (*guṇa*) of energy.

"Objective reality" requires one to acknowledge one's state, wherever one finds oneself, with one's anxieties, agitation, and suffering. This simple act will create a stop (*nirodha*) in the mechanical flow, and open up a conscious and impersonal space in which phenomena are perceived differently, with more freedom and less conditioning, and without the subjective interference of the person. When I begin to be alert and totally attentive, a space of benevolent peace opens up for each activity of my daily life, in which the desire for a result and projections fade out, and give way to the action taking place, here and now. I can interact with the world with full awareness, and because I am forewarned and aware of the mental processes at work at the heart of the action; I can remain tranquil without necessarily reacting to mental or emotional mechanisms, or to the stimuli detected by the senses. This quality of presence to one's own manifestation, both inner and outer, and this alert observation of one's own thoughts, words, and deeds, is the point of entry into the practice. This first verse alone says it all. The following verse shows how to recognize this Presence, by removing the phenomena that veil it.

योगश्चित्तवृत्तनिरोधः॥२॥
Yogaścittavṛttinirodhaḥ||2||

2. Yoga is the stopping (*nirodha*) of the fluctuations (*vṛtti*) of the mind (*citta*).

The Sanskrit term *nirodha* means "restriction, restraint, repression, stopping, interruption, removal, ending, or suspension." Let us understand from the outset that by "suspension" or "stopping" of thought (*citta*), we are not talking about it disappearing completely, in the sense that it no longer exists. It is rather about a process of disidentification in which thought is perceived as an object, a mere event or a phenomenon, to be welcomed with kindness and without grasping, in the space of Awareness. Nothing is repressed; on the contrary, everything finds its place in this welcoming space, which remains unaffected by what is taking place in it, and acts with equanimity toward everything.

The Buddha himself used this word *nirodha* to designate his third Noble Truth (*āryasatya*) about the end of suffering (*duḥkha-nirodhaḥ*). The ancient Greeks used the term *epoché* (ἐποχή or *epokhē*) meaning "stopping, suspension, or ending." About the same time as Patañjali, but in Greece, the philosopher Sextus Empiricus spoke about it in the following manner: "'Suspense' is a state of mental rest owing to which we neither deny nor affirm anything. 'Quietude' is an untroubled and tranquil condition of soul." (*Outlines of Pyrrhonism,* 1.10). Almost two thousand years later, Western philosophy, quoting Husserl, defined it as the suspension or the "bracketing" of judgment, and thus of thought, which itself is the very tool of judgment. An Indian, a Greek, and a Frenchman certainly have different thought content, but when their thoughts stop, all their functions stop, and the Reality that remains is identical for each one of them. There is no distinction, no difference, no boundary, no him, no them, and no me. There is only that which is: yoga or Oneness. All content, including the notions of subject and object, and all thought functions (the mind, the sense of "me," the intellect, and memory) are dissolved in the pure and nondual Awareness; even the thought "OM=mc². " Everything dissolves, even the notion and the act of suspending. Everything becomes peaceful, shuts down, is wiped out, and disappears (*nirvāṇa*) into Awareness. And being well established in its nature (*svarūpa*), the being experiences supreme bliss, free of the changes inherent to phenomena.

But this spontaneous and absolute recognition, although seemingly evident, is quite rare. By extension, from a relative point of view, the *sūtra* teaches us that yoga, as a means, consists in observing and coordinating the mental flow with awareness, so that thoughts serve us instead of enslaving us. Patañjali uses the word *citta* to designate thought as a whole, with all its functions. The word *vṛtti* signifies the automatic mechanisms, conditioned modifications, fluctuations, changes, and forms of the mental field. The word *nirodha,* in a broad sense, is another way of apprehending and engaging with the manifestation of thoughts, with the manner in which the object of one's experience takes form, in phenomenological terms. The perception of the peripheral movements reinforces the awareness of the still center, which reveals itself when they calm down.

There is nothing to remove or annihilate except this defective perception, due to which I take myself to be what I am not. As for the rest, everything is useful, including thoughts, when they are calm, observed, and totally in sync with the breath, the body, the sensations, and the surrounding environment. One must observe, allow the clouds of desire to float by, and allow the river of life to flow in the space of Awareness, without grasping or seizing, without holding onto anything, so as to remain effortlessly in the conscious Source. The practice is a phenomenological reduction, a conversion of the gaze that enables one to transcend the veils of ignorance (the defective perception) by bringing the attention back, prior to the flow of mental projections.

Patañjali then describes the attitudes that allow one to cultivate this quality of equanimity in the face of the desire and aversion that agitate the mind, strengthen attachment, and condition destiny.

This *sūtra* is applicable to all paths that recommend being fully aware of sensations and thoughts. The methods or forms of yoga may vary, and are adapted to one's abilities and maturity, but the required effort and the goal are the same. The mind's activity can be controlled or stopped in different ways:

> When it is stopped through the alert observation of thoughts and the discrimination of their different functions, the very act of observation will calm down the mind and stop its activities.
>
> Or the mind's activity can be stopped through reduction and the search for the source of the mind (*vicāra*).
>
> Or it can be stopped through concentration on one single thought, in order to reduce the others and make them dissolve into one thought alone, which itself will end up disappearing in the quietude of pure awareness (*yoga*).
>
> The mind's activity can also be stopped through the control and stopping of breath alone (*prāṇayāma*).
>
> Or through the careful combination of poses, breaths, gestures, locks, and concentrations (*haṭhayoga*); through conscious sleep (*yoganidrā*), and in numerous other ways, be they conscious, useless, or accidental. All attempts share the same goal.

No matter what I am doing or which approach I choose, attention, self-observation, and the inquiry into "who" is doing something (or not), are important. The energy of the inquiry thus initiates a dynamic that awakens me to the mystery, which I cannot describe, but which I discover as being the most essential space of this mystery that I am.

तदा द्रष्टुः स्वरूपेऽवस्थानम्॥ ३॥
Tadā draṣṭuḥ svarūpe'vasthānam ||3||

3. Then (*tadā*), the witness (*draṣṭuḥ*) is established (*avasthānam*) in its essential nature (*svarūpe*).

Draṣṭuḥ (from the term *drsh*, which means "to see") is "the one who sees," the witness. When thought is suspended, the Self, firmly established in itself, is revealed. The witness of thoughts is revealed in its true nature, which is formless and which contains all appearing and disappearing forms. Attention awakens to its own essence: Awareness becomes aware of itself. The being is known as pure joy without object, like a Vision without a seer and without any object being seen. A crystal takes on the color of the objects it is placed on, but in reality, it is colorless and free of the colors appearing in it. But this impersonal seeing can neither be described nor explained, and it can neither be developed nor thought about, because it exists prior to the mind and cannot be defined or grasped. Remaining in its original nature (*svarūpe*), staying in it, and residing firmly in itself (*avasthāna*), it is like the sun that continues to shine even when the clouds cover it. But for the one who has never seen the sun, the clouds must first move away, even if only for a moment, for one to see its brilliance, feel its warmth, and bathe in its light. Once again, this is just another image that may veil the presence and splendor of the sun of Awareness. It is like a vast ocean taking itself to be a small wave, which, sooner or later, will break down and disappear, or remember that it is the eternal ocean, and not just a small ripple. Different experiences play out on a tranquil and unchanging background, in the peaceful center that observes the peripheral movements, observing without getting involved. If Patañjali does not say much more about this Life within life, it is because the only way to understand the living Vision in a lasting manner is to experience it for oneself. The Sanskrit term for suffering is *duḥkhā,* which literally means "to be badly centered," and the term *sukhā,* meaning "to be well centered," is used to designate happiness. Very clearly, the problem arises due to identification with the different states of the mind, which make one off-centered; and this is explained in the following aphorism.

वृत्तिसारूप्यमितरत्र॥४॥

Vṛttisārūpyamitaratra ||4||

4. Otherwise (*itaratra*), there is identification (*sārūpyam*)
with the fluctuation (*vṛtti*) of thoughts.

This *sūtra* summarizes the whole human condition and the origin of its suffering, by directly pointing to the root of the problem, which is identification. The term *sārūpya* literally means "to have the same form as." It designates similarity or resemblance, or being the image of something. When the subject takes himself or herself to be the object he or she is looking at, there is identification. The Self, identified with thoughts, takes itself to be these thoughts, and thinks, "I think, therefore I am." The formless takes itself to be the forms appearing in it. It is only when identification ceases, by means of the suspension of thoughts, that the Self recognizes itself by itself. And that is yoga, as defined by traditional Indian philosophy. The approach then takes on many forms. The manifold is born from Oneness.

Yoga is both the means and the end leading to this. As a means, it consists in an integral education of the body and the mind, which is mainly a preparation or readiness for something. But if this seems simple, it does not mean that it is easy. Letting go of something requires one to know well what one is holding on to, and especially to know who is holding on to it. In other words, the most important thing is to correctly observe with alertness these fluctuations of the mind (*vṛtti*) with which an individual is constantly identified. Otherwise, we risk living unaware in our cave, behaving mechanically, inventing sciences that are but the ruin of the soul, like a puppet whose strings are being pulled by life's uncertainties.

So, what is this object that it is so hard to let go of? What does Patañjali mean by fluctuations (*vṛtti*), or by thoughts (*citta*)? Can I truly recognize them? With which tools? Can thoughts decide to stop by themselves? And if not, then how can they stop? *Vṛtti* literally designates "movement, flow, transformation, or behavior"; in philosophy, we speak of the fluctuation of thoughts (*cittavṛtti*). In the next seven aphorisms (from 5 to 11), Patañjali enumerates five modalities of thought.

When the changing flow of phenomena is trying to steal one's attention, Awareness seems to be reduced to names, forms, and appearances, as if the vast sky were reduced to a mere cloud, or as if gold were reduced to a mere ornament, or as if a crystal thinks it is green because it is lying on the grass. We seek permanent happiness outside ourselves, in ephemeral phenomena that we do not even take the time to observe, and we end up losing ourselves before we disappear completely. Instead, we can observe that which does not change and listen to that which remains still and silent, behind the noisy and agitated forms of thought, which Patañjali later describes. The more we identify with thoughts, emotions, and sensations, the more we are attached to the image we have of ourselves, and the greater the reaction of suffering will be. Sensations and emotions are neither bad nor to be repressed. The whole problem comes from the fact that we think of thoughts, emotions, and sensations as belonging to someone, to "me." Or from the belief that the moon is moving when we perceive its reflection moving on the surface of water.

The philosophy of nondualism (*advaita-vedānta*) points directly to the "I"-thought (*aham-vṛtti* or *ahaṃkāra*) as being the root cause of all suffering. In deep sleep, the sense of "me" disappears; nothing is held onto, thus leaving room for the peace of non-knowing. When one wakes up, the fluctuation of the "I"-thought brings with it the whole phenomenal world, and the suffering inherent to it. Simply being aware of this process brings about a trembling of one's whole being, suspending all possibility of thought. During this pause, it may be possible to recognize a particular stillness, which is tranquil, from which I then begin to live, intermittently in the beginning, and then in a more stable and continuous manner, allowing it to calmly illuminate the world.

If Husserl described the Buddha as a super phenomenologist, the same can be said for Patañjali. He went far beyond a mere description of phenomena and his work invites us to verify its authenticity by ourselves. Between two thoughts, between two fluctuations, between two states, I can immediately know the taste of the link, the flavor of *yoga* (literally meaning "to harness"), and of the common substance that underlines these different phenomena. Moreover, in the here and now (*sūtra* I.1), I can proceed by becoming aware of the phenomena, according to the process of systematic reduction, which consists in bringing the attention back to myself, in order to allow the different structures of the being to reveal themselves. I can transcend them (I.2) until I recognize the still witness (I.3) prior to the moving phenomena, the silent essence hidden beneath the sensitive aspect of sound, of the body, and of the noisy mind, without identifying with their form and movement, without believing myself to be every phenomena that appears in Awareness and without saying "me" or "mine" (I.4).

Without Presence, I am just projecting an image of the world; whereas in reality, it is simply manifesting in Awareness, which is free of the fluctuations and flow of the mind, and of the waves of thought. The path toward this Awareness, and its recognition, are simultaneously the meaning, the aim, and the nature of yoga. But if this realization opens up to the Absolute, it is not an end in itself; it is also an art of living, which can only be integrated in my ordinary daily life through practice, continuous daily training (*sādhana*), and conscious repetition.

When my false identities are suspended, the recognition of the Self is intimately felt through the different layers that veil the pure being, by allowing a peace, which vibrates in all cells of the body, to descend upon them (I.3). But, most of the time, we are identified with these false identities, and we live, blinded and asleep, in what Husserl calls the "natural attitude," or what Plato calls the "cave," like puppets whose strings are being pulled by the automatic and changing phenomena of life. Cutting the strings of conditioning and awakening to pure Awareness is the meaning of yoga.

Yoga invites one to recognize how Awareness observes everything through the intellect, the mind, the senses, and the body. The phenomena are reflected on it, like on a screen, and identification consists in mistaking the screen for the images, or the sky for the cloud passing through. A movement of thought thinks "me" or "mine," and I hold onto different things, thinking, "I am this or that." This veils my true nature and makes me forget it. I cannot access this essential nature; I can only make an effort to remove the obstacle preventing me from doing so. The recognition itself is spontaneous and effortless.

And yet, the sages of ancient India declare that yoga is deep contemplation, pure attention, and awareness without object (*yoga-samādhi*). This Presence must first reveal itself through the attentive observation of phenomena with equanimity, and through phenomenological reduction and inner investigation. Once "what it is not" is perceived (everything appears and disappears in it), what remains is "what it is," without effort; it is thus recognized in its essential nature (*svarūpa*). This is often experienced as an awakening or a realization.

However, such a realization can be rapidly overtaken by the force of attraction of mental fluctuations, and projected in the agitated world of phenomena through identification. The practice of reduction subsequently consists in coming back to what is, by using discrimination, and by bringing the attention back to its ever-peaceful and joyous source, in which all phenomena are reflected and welcomed with effortless benevolence. The word *yoga* designates union or Oneness, the conscious effort to recognize, bring together, conciliate, and coordinate that which seems multiple and dispersed. The recognition arises as a result of the long work of integration in all aspects of life, which becomes serene, balanced, harmonious, and reconciled under this nondual gaze that effortlessly embraces the old and the new, and the joys and the sorrows. It will descend into each layer of the being and permeate it with its vitality and joy, going into the cells, which are full of awareness. Integration consists in cultivating this witness state, this phenomenological attitude, and this quality of total awareness of every thought, word, or gesture, until one is firmly established in the Self, in the unwavering bliss of the being, internally free of phenomena and suffering.

No matter what I or you think about this, all these thoughts and judgments only appear and disappear within this Awareness, without ever affecting it, while it remains without judgment and discrimination, and benevolent to all that takes place in it. The Awareness gives us everything, but we are too encumbered to receive it. This is when the practice of yoga, as defined by Patañjali, as a practice of Presence, resolutely phenomenological, conscious, and contemplative, can help us to leave room for this bliss of the being, in the very tumult of ordinary activities.

From the outset, Patañjali gives us the key that will open all doors. Pointing directly to the root of the problem, he invites us to immediately dive into the Absolute, so as to bring the attention back to the relative phenomena, and allow for the observation of the mechanisms of manifestation; the action of suspension thus allows for observing as if it were the first time, without bias or knowledge. If all this seems too complicated for the mind, this new outlook on the world, which no longer passes through the prism of the associative and ordinary mind, will make the approach of reduction and the return to this essential Vision easier. It will no longer be regarded as an effort, but as an energy, which continuously underlines rest and emptiness, quietude and joy of being.

May we thus be sufficiently empty, until we are nothing at all, and recognize this joyful Awareness that is always full!

An Approach to Indian Psychology

*A Phenomenological Reflection on the Nature
and Functions of Thought*

The sustained observation of phenomena can gradually lead to a phenomenological reflection on the nature and functions of thought, based on Indian psychology, which constitutes the foundation of these practices. Thus, thought, as a whole, is seen as an "internal organ" that perceives external objects through the five sense organs and acts upon them through the five organs of action. This "internal organ," the thoughts or the mind, exercises four important functions, allowing for knowledge about external objects and intellectual activity. Let us call them the mind, the ego, the intellect, and the unconscious; and let us remember that they are all composed of thoughts.

The mind consists of thoughts and sensory impressions, like the body consists of foods and vital air. It receives external stimuli through the five senses of perception, which create a constantly changing state of thoughts. The mind feels emotions and it guides, supervises, or connects with the functioning of the senses, like the reins linking the horses (the senses) to the coachman (the intellect). The mind reacts by feeling desire or aversion, according to the sensory impressions that are received. The mental formations happen mechanically, stemming from raw data. When the senses are no longer pulled outward, but withdrawn like a turtle, pulled back from the mind, the latter generates dreams and thoughts, which feed on the impressions relative to the dream itself or on the force of impressions that emerge from the unconscious, and which condition or color dreams and thoughts, reasoning, memory, and imagination. Always in motion, the mind doubts and believes, and oscillates between desire and fear.

While being linked with the mind—albeit "closer" to awareness as its direct reflection—*the intellect* exercises a different function, related to knowledge, discrimination, determination, will, and judgment, as well as intuition. The intellect receives the light of awareness and reflects it by illuminating the mind. It analyzes, decides, makes its choices, and formulates grand ideas, according to the impressions that have already been automatically sorted out by the mind. Intellect decides which response to send back to a stimulus. But it is still comprised of thoughts and conditioned desires, most of the time stifled by the agitated movements of the mind and the outflow of the unconscious. It plays a part in the simple awareness of being, without the identity of "I" because its function is, by nature, impersonal.

The unconscious exercises a function related to memory; to a certain extent, it belongs to the intellect. Together, they constitute "individual awareness," which illuminates agitation and the sense of "me." It may appear to be individual and limited when it is identified with the mind and the ego, and when it functions through them. The unconscious stores memories about past experiences in a dormant or underlying form, or in the form of unmanifested tendencies, and it refreshes them in the mind as memories, habits, biases, and representations. When one calls on one's memory, one solicits this function. The unconscious is characterized by an absence of suffering, like in deep sleep, during which everything is withdrawn into this function where the senses are silent. The recollection of dormant impressions stored here determines and conditions the nature of the intellect, the mind, and actions, in a mechanical way, by reinforcing the sense of "me" based on habits and memory.

It is not surprising that the unconscious belongs to what Indian philosophy calls the "causal body," because it causes or produces thoughts, and influences them constantly. In the natural attitude of ordinary awareness, when the intellect is not alert, the voices and habits of the unconscious lead the mind to act in the world, in a way that is not necessarily adapted to the circumstances. The intellect should be making these decisions, but when it is stifled by agitation, the mind only receives the orders of the memories and patterns of habits, also colored by the ego's desires and aversions, and the totality of impressions related to past experiences, stored in the unconscious in a dormant form.

Lastly, *the ego* is simply the function that creates the sense of "me" or the "I-thought," or the "me and mine": the process of individuation itself. It is the thought of being a separate entity, limited to the body-mind structure, an ego-thought that only exists with reference to the past, to memories and habits, and that only manifests when mental agitation, the intellect, and the entire body-mind structure coexist. It is, in a manner of speaking, the reflection of the being or pure Awareness in any thought apparatus. A sensation, a feeling, or a thought of being, the sense of "I," are only the pale reflection of the Awareness itself. Ego does not exist by itself; it is just a reaction, a strain that disappears when the tension is released. But it seems to be present when awareness is not, like the empty sky seems to disappear when it is filled with big clouds. This function claims authorship of everything, and leads one to believe, albeit wrongly, that it is Awareness itself; when, in reality, it is nothing but a thought or a simple event, which is at the source of several woes and therefore, of suffering. Sages recommend the path of action to eradicate it, which consists in selfless service, being present to the action performed without projecting its result; it also includes the awareness of having the opportunity to act now in the best manner possible, but without being able to control the result of those actions, which depend on external phenomena and diverse laws. The path of love, devotion, and kindness to all beings also allows for setting oneself aside for the benefit of others.

The path of knowledge, which is resolutely phenomenological, encourages one to discriminate between the real (permanent), the noumenon so to speak, and the unreal (impermanent), meaning the world of phenomena. It can be summed up in the continuous and reductive search of the Self, of Awareness, through the constant investigation about the nature of the one who is operating: who am I? To whom do these thoughts appear? Who is thinking? Who is afraid? Who dies? Who is meditating? And so on. The energy used by the investigation, being unable to formulate an answer, withdraws from the ego-questioner and interrupts it, weakens it, and dissolves it, thus revealing the unreal nature of the interdependent, impermanent, and impersonal phenomenon. Regardless of the answer or impression provoked, it is only a passing and ephemeral mental or emotional event, which comes and goes in the impersonal space of Awareness.

For example, when I see another being, when he or she enters my field of vision, what happens? It is clear that the eye perceives the shapes and colors and sends the raw information to the mind, which can doubt what is being presented to it (who is it?). Helped by memory, the mind recognizes the person, and the intellect states, "It's Sandrine," whereas the ego thinks, "I know her, she's my sister, my friend, my wife, me, my, mine, and so on" or "I recognize her," and so on.

All this happens too quickly for ordinary awareness, and seems to manifest as one single movement. But sustained contemplation shows that the process obeys a precise and completely automatic sequence, in the form of vibrations or rapid waves, which are changing and are linked to one another by relations of cause and effect, or of phenomena conditioning conditioned phenomena. Thus, one can differentiate between the vibrations of the mind and the vibrations of the intellect, the unconscious, or the ego.

Suppose you were to carelessly pick up a burning hot cup of tea, and you let go of it immediately with a squeal. What happened in that split-second? Several phenomena succeeded one another. When your hand (the organ of action) touched the hot cup, your skin (the sense organ) transported the stimulus of heat to the mind, thus forcing the intellect to evaluate and determine the appropriate kind of response. Helped by the memory of past experiences (the impressions left by the experience of being burnt), the intellect orders the mind, more or less precisely, to react, by transmitting orders to the body via the brain and the central nervous system. Thus, in the cited example, the intellect, helped by the memory, commands the hand to be removed so as to not be burned.

Perhaps I am watching a film, a thriller, with a lot of suspense. The vibrations of the mind are activated. When a mystery needs to be solved, the intellect begins to vibrate for thinking, analyzing, and discriminating, which erases, or at least reduces, the mental vibration. The intellect reflects on the data collected by the mind during the film, while the unconscious stores and keeps the memory of information and impressions. The ego is happy to react and assumes the role of the one who perceives, feels, thinks, reflects, and remembers. But all these functions are only aspects of one sole organ of thought. Being fully aware of these vibrations and movements, of their manifestation and disappearance, shows that Awareness is always present, with or without thought, in the states of waking, dreaming, and deep sleep, like the thread present at the heart of every pearl in a necklace.

The phenomena are only reflected in Awareness, like images in a mirror. Whether there is a face or not, a thought or not, the mirror remains in its own nature, unaffected by what it reflects. This realization can surface in the space between two thoughts or two states, in the underlying silence that unites them, also recognized as the reality in which these thoughts occur. It is the realization that the sun still shines behind the clouds, whether they are big or small, black or white; and the reality that I am is not affected by what is taking place in it. Recognizing this is truly liberating, and self-observation is the royal path to this realization.

When I repeat a word with full awareness, what are the processes involved? The intellect decides to chant "I" while inhaling, and "Am" while exhaling, concentrating on the repetition. Gradually, a space opens up, in a manner of speaking, between the intellect repeating the words and the witness aware of this repetition. The word-thought is reabsorbed in this silent space, like a mass of undifferentiated Awareness. And presto, the mental vibration has taken over again, reinforced by the advent of thoughts coloring it, making a flow of thoughts appear, which take me far away from the repetition, as I identify with and am carried away by peripheral movements. Suddenly, like a flash, there is awareness of this distraction, followed by a moment of suspension, an interval, a space between two vibrations. Then, helped by the memory, the intellect takes control of the repetition once again.

I notice, at the same time, that when I try to remember something, I cannot remember it, or I cannot find the answer. Suddenly, the thinking stops, it is dissolved in a kind of emptiness or tranquil unawareness, from which the memory emerges, spontaneously and effortlessly. The phenomenon of memory is thus perceptible during meditation, which breaks down the barriers between what is normally called conscious and unconscious, throwing light on the whole inner organ, and not only on the visible tip of the iceberg. By concentrating on the breath and on a word or a phrase, with my eyes shut, my attention turns inward, and a withdrawal of the senses operates. Thus, deprived of the constant flow of sensory impressions induced by contact with the external world, the mind, finding itself with less food, will keep going back to feed on the reserves of impressions stored in the unconscious. Cut off from the abundance of external impressions, the mind will draw on the reserves of the unconscious, which begin to surface.

In this manner, after a distinct moment of silence, the thoughts resurface with force, as if propelled by the unconscious, creating pleasant or unpleasant sensations in the body. If I react to these sensations with desire or aversion, I produce new impressions of desire and aversion, which are added to the already existing supply, and which condition my present and future mechanical thoughts. Thus, the more I react, the more the mind stirs up, and I gather more and more memories of reactions; and this makes me react even more, as I repeat the same conditioned patterns over and over again.

On the other hand, if I do not react with desire or aversion when a thought arises or a sensation appears, I create neither agitation nor suffering; I do not produce new impressions to replenish the stock; but above all, I notice that the supply is gradually beginning to run out, and this brings a unique feeling of lightness and joy. While practicing, as well as in daily life, the moments of silence will become longer, more profound, and more frequent. Regular training is like a fast for the mind, which will eventually allow for a glimpse of pure Awareness. And in the same manner, it is from this silent unawareness that important ideas, premonitions, and intuition emerge. Reality is directly perceived, without the ordinary prism of the mind.

Actually, it is also from this unawareness that the sense of "me" emerges, in the transition between sleeping and waking. The intellect wakes up and comes into contact with the mind, making the "I-thought" appear. During this brief pause, it is possible to recognize the underlying reality that connects both states, as well as both movements of thoughts. With the "I-thought," the mind's world resurfaces and the phenomenal world manifests once again. Conversely, when one falls asleep, the senses, the mind, the sense of "me," followed by the intellect, are dissolved in the unawareness of deep and peaceful sleep.

Similarly, by practicing the repetition of a word, without any kind of expectation, or simply by observing the flow of thoughts, the mind and the sense of "me" withdraw into the intellect, which in turn withdraws into the conscious bliss of non-knowing, where memories remain dormant. It is here, closest to that which is nevertheless everywhere, that the miracle of Awareness can take place, far from all ordinary intentions. But at this stage, there is nobody trying to attain a target. That being said, when, by grace or by accident, the arrow of attention awakens to its own substance by turning toward itself, it then realizes that it is no more different from the target than the ability to burn is from fire. The being is simply reflected in its own Awareness and joy of being, enjoying its freedom, and untouched by any condition. In this vision or pure attention, there is neither a subject, nor an object, nor a witness who observes, nor an object that is being observed, but only pure unified Awareness, in which "All is One." This is also what important spiritual traditions call "Love."

Self-Observation and
Total Awareness
in Daily Life

No matter whether you are sitting, standing, lying down, or moving around, in any pose or in any situation, the contemplation of thoughts is the royal path to deep-seated peace. Contemplation does not replace any other activity; it can simply be added on, or rather, it recognizes itself in the common substratum or in the silent background of every activity. It is effortless. It requires nothing more than to welcome that which is presenting itself. Of course, by observing a sensation, which is the foundation of the practice, I can observe the psychophysical mechanics as a whole, because everything is connected.

To help in this realization, the guidance of a teacher can evoke specific images conducive to the revelation, as it is customary to do in the nondualistic approaches in Indian philosophy. I can notice thoughts, or a series of thoughts, like soap bubbles, ribbons, flowing streams or a river, ocean waves, clouds in the sky, or like a movie projected on a screen, formless and silent in Awareness. These currents or this flow of thoughts merge, collide with one another, nourish and condition each other, more or less quickly, and with more or less agitation. The perception of a thought reinforces the awareness of the unconscious, and of the Awareness itself.

The act of tranquil contemplation awakens to the pure vision of the being, also recognizable between two thoughts or two states (as in the case of waking and sleep, or the other way around). In this pure vision, thoughts are merely events, changing mental phenomena that are conditioned by dormant memories, which appear and disappear. Perceived by an impersonal gaze that is vaster, and seen for what they really are, these thoughts lose their power of attraction and of fascination, and begin to serve the individual rather than enslave him or her. In this vision, in this space of Awareness, the slightest agitation is immediately detected, and as a consequence, the agitation is effortlessly dissolved in the conscious vision. This does not require any particular technique or action; on the contrary, the intention itself only constitutes a mental event. This pure listening is not within the scope of an individual; nobody can do it, because it is the person—as a body-mind structure or as a phenomena—who is seen and observed, with his or her grand and small ideas, with his or her biases, judgments, opinions, intentions, and other claims, which are merely thoughts, or with his or her emotions, which are just the body's reactions to the mind.

In this pure listening, there is nothing to do, because nothing can be done. The very idea of doing, or of being someone who is doing something, is still just a thought. This listening consists in an attitude that holds onto nothing, acts with equanimity, and is non-dual, in which there is nothing to grasp or to repress. The listening is only the return to the listening itself, the withdrawal of awareness into itself, the awakening of the sky to itself, by itself, spontaneously and effortlessly. The thought, or the feeling of "me" or "I," is just another event emerging and disappearing in this reality, which is a living void, full of the phenomenal world. But this distinction between subject and object is merely intellectual and conceptual. For, in awareness, everything is One. There is no inner and outer, and therefore, the invitation in the beginning to "go into oneself" is only a mental phrase intended for the mind. If Awareness is already everywhere, to where can I withdraw?

This essential recognition is not an act of concentration either, which is still an effort, but rather a kind of expansion and complete openness, unconditioned and without origin. It is what is, that which remains the same no matter what state the body-mind structure finds itself in, be it in the state of waking, dreaming, or sleep, whether thoughts are calm or agitated, right or wrong. All phenomena surface from this conscious source, the integrating force of the different structures of the being and other phenomena, somewhat like a mother, like the matrix in which everything manifests, unfolds, interacts, changes, and is dissolved, including the concept of time and space. It is not about reflecting either, but rather about observing when the concept and the very act of conceptualizing present themselves to awareness.

This contemplation on the play of the elements and of the energy takes place spontaneously in awareness. The wheel of thoughts, words, and deeds, the wheel of destiny, turns in the space of Awareness. This is why daily practice, which concerns each and every moment, does not require seizing the wheel in order to change it, stop it, or make it go faster or slower. Instead it is recognizing oneself as the space of pure openness, in the contemplation of the wheel turning at its own natural pace, without grasping anything. Even the desire to attain something belongs to the realm of the wheel in motion, because it is also seen, as it manifests and disappears spontaneously. Therefore, there is nothing to attain or become, the "subtler" or so-called "advanced" states still only involve the person. It is simply about being, empty of opinions and beliefs, biases and judgments, and becoming aware of the absolute freedom hidden beneath the sensitive aspect of automatic phenomena.

This is why pure and real contemplation cannot be qualified as good or bad, or positive or negative, simply because these dualistic concepts still belong to thought, and they come and go in thought itself. It is not about wanting to contemplate either, because this desire also belongs to the person. Contemplation is happening. Whether I know it or not, I am seen. But, distracted by the flow of automatic thoughts, I identify with them and fail to recognize that which truly sees. Not only do I not recognize it, I claim authorship of it, thinking that it is "me" who is doing it. All this is still just the play of the elements.

Therefore, the only thing to "do" is to remain quiet, in the listening and with effortless openness, without any tension. If the thought "I am contemplating" or "I am practicing" emerges in Awareness, I allow it to manifest and disappear, noticing that this "I" is not meditating, but in fact, is simply passing through the empty space of contemplation. Simply noticing and becoming aware of the fact that I am still trying to control it, brings me back to pure contemplation without holding onto anything. When I try to be calm, I am only nourishing a thought that will not really calm me down. As soon as this contemplation seems to require an effort of any kind, or causes any kind of strain, it means that a movement of the mind has overtaken it. It is just like the feeling that it is "me" who is contemplating. As a result of seeing that this feeling also comes and goes, it is identified as a mere phenomenon, and the belief in the "me" contemplating gradually crumbles, leaving room for an impersonal presence, in which I can recognize myself as ever-peaceful, blissful, and unchanging.

Every opportunity offered to us should be considered as a chance to remind us of this natural recognition, not "natural" in the sense that Husserl evokes, whereby raw material must be worked on and made to evolve, but rather "natural" in the sense of an original and essential reality, which is perfect by nature. Subsequently, the force of repetition allows for the integration and reconciliation of these seemingly dualistic relations: illuminated by the understanding of this new outlook, free of everything, one learns again how to live in harmony with oneself and with one's environment, aware of wholeness that is constantly fragmented by the blind belief in an all-powerful "me." The pull of identification, which is repeatedly exposed, begins to gradually lose its grip.

Let us illustrate this with a theatrical metaphor. Pierre is an actor playing the role of Hamlet; he is so committed to his role that he takes himself to be Hamlet, and completely identifies with him. Suddenly, Pierre remembers that he is not Hamlet, but Pierre playing the role of Hamlet. But he does not recognize, even for a minute, that he is also playing another role: that of being completely identified with Pierre, who he believes exists. By becoming aware that he is no more Pierre than he is Hamlet, that he is no more than another observer of this situation, something very tangible seems to happen. There is still nothing to gain, but there is an immense joy emerging from that which disappears, namely the fear of death and of being nothing.

This also concerns the greed for having certain experiences, which takes me away, every single time, from the empty obviousness, dragging me yet again to the periphery of the being. Changing and short-lived experiences only have meaning in their manifestation, because as soon as they disappear, they are no more than memories, which means they are no more than thoughts. But no matter which phenomenon emerges, it always emerges in this timeless and formless space. The center of the wheel is static, but it is the space in which and through which everything takes place. Whether the wheel is in motion or at a standstill, this empty center remains as it is, unaffected by change.

So what is needed is to stop wanting to pause the wheel of time and existence, but rather let it be what it is, aware that the very desire to stop it only feeds its dynamic of movement. It is the mind itself, which is trying to stop the mind; by making a move to stop it, it only keeps going, in one big endless circle. But if I just remain present, as awareness, as the witness of the circle, I can recognize myself as the conscious and impersonal space in which the circle itself is seen. And if I try, as an individual, to attain this awareness, to come back to it or to remain in it, it will only be another phenomenon perceived in the space of Awareness, by the Awareness itself. All the more reason to stay quiet and let life be, allowing one's practice and daily activities to unfold spontaneously, free of the burden of desire, aversion, and expectations, in the joy inherent to the now.

Awareness Is Always
on Vacation

It is important to recognize that, very often, most people tend to confuse Awareness with thought. This confusion is the consequence of the identification with phenomena that emerge in Awareness. In my ordinary state, I do not even realize that I am identified with and take myself to be everything that manifests; I do not even realize that I am unaware of everything that is happening in me, all the time. In this state, I only react to external circumstances like a puppet whose strings are being pulled by the automatic phenomena of existence. I unconsciously believe myself to be an object tossed around by the agitated course of daily life. Every feeling, every emotion, and every thought says "me" or "I," without any discrimination. I am living in a cave and taking the shadows to be real, and I suffer because of this suffering, again and again.

Then, one day, the practice, work on oneself, begins. I start to become aware of phenomena and discover a new quality of rest and relaxation. I become a little more attentive to what is happening in "me." But, due to unawareness, I am still convinced that I will find happiness and Self-Realization in these phenomena. So I try to induce them, hold on to them, transform them, choose them, or chase them away, without realizing that this only constitutes another automatic reaction, which continues to pull at me, and continues to feed this process of reacting to desire and aversion, to small joys and moments of sadness, to pain and suffering. I continue to "like" and "dislike," believing that I will find lasting happiness in phenomena that are only passing through and taking everything along; I continue to believe that one day, some time in the future, in space and time, I will have a particular experience that will make me another person than the one I already am.

I read in a book that one must "practice, practice, and practice more," and that the "repetition" will bring about the much longed-for "change." This seems logical, insofar as I have always been taught that one must make an effort to obtain something in return. This idea gives me incentive, and I enthusiastically take up my practice again, only to be discouraged once more. This can go on for one's whole life, a situation that is uncomfortable and hard to live with. And all this time, I remain convinced that I will obtain this "transformation" only through great efforts, and as a consequence, I will suffer even more, because I will not succeed in this endeavor. It is indeed exhausting to run after oneself, or to chase Awareness or happiness, without ever being able to catch up with it.

From the very beginning, the problem comes from the fact that "I" want to "change myself," when I do not even know who this "me," having this desire, really is. I neither know this "I" claiming to operate, nor the object being changed. But, fueled by imagination and instilled beliefs, I begin to practice, and think that I am progressing or I am not sure what else. And naturally, I continue to suffer, to struggle and fight.

This is the right moment to stop, and simply become aware of one's general state, without trying to change or transform anything. This in itself is enough. Just observe the tensions in the body and the mind, quietly and with attention. Simply welcome the phenomena as they manifest in Awareness, without bias, and without trying to attain a particular state. Just be aware of your state, of your different states, of the transition from one state to another, from one thought to another. Relax in this presence that is observing. Who is observing? "Me!" "I!" "The presence!" "The witness!" "I am the witness!" and so on. Here, it is essential to see that all these answers are only thoughts appearing and disappearing in Awareness, like clouds passing in the sky. "I am the sky!" is still just a thought. Let it go. Stay as the pure welcoming space.

While observing phenomena, I do realize that, as a result of some efforts, I can indeed influence the body (by practicing sports, for example) and the mind (by reading books, following training programs, learning new things, collecting information, learning to concentrate, and so on). All these activities are interesting, inspiring even, but by no means will they help me to know Awareness. All these activities, and thoughts about these activities, come and go in Awareness. Who am I? "Awareness!"—just another thought.

By remaining as the one who observes, without trying to interfere or to concentrate, without any intention other than silently observing what manifests at every moment, the flame of attention, which is impersonal, illuminates all phenomena, and thus begins to awaken to its own substance. Awareness, which until now was always aware of an object, thus begins to awaken to itself, by itself. I am no longer this or that; I am no longer a person experiencing something in particular; I AM, simply. Not a thought, a feeling or a sensation of being, but Being itself, in which all phenomena manifest. The attention with which I recognize this being is the same attention with which this impersonal Awareness of Being knows me, as a body-mind structure manifesting as thoughts, words, and actions.

I cannot grasp this intellectually, but I can accept that I do not understand it. Awareness is not an object. And the so-called subject is just another thought. A new quality of tranquility emerges. I cannot explain the mystery of Awareness; nor do I know anything about it, nor can I say anything about it. And yet, failing to explain what it is, I may be given the opportunity to recognize that I am it, I am the mystery. I cannot know it, but I can recognize it, and I can see that both the knowing and the non-knowing are just states of thought appearing and disappearing in Awareness, which always remains unaffected by what is taking place in it. The body and thoughts are changing, in time and in space, but Awareness remains the ever-peaceful background of all experiences, whether they are good or bad.

Awareness is always available, open, full of life, and welcoming all phenomena, states, and events, without exception. The slightest intention or effort to do or act on something is, yet again, just a phenomenon. "I" cannot welcome anything. The feeling of welcoming something is also a phenomenon. There is welcoming, an openness aware of itself. Welcoming, but nobody to do it. Awareness is always free or vacant, open wide, and always on vacation (from the word *vacare,* which means "to be empty"). So then why strive to make all these efforts? Why not just rest in Awareness, which is always resting, always on vacation?

Several centuries ago, an Indian sage wrote "the one who simply abides in Awareness, and detaches oneself from the identification with the body, will, in this very moment, become happy, peaceful, and free from bondage." (*Aṣṭāvakra-Gītā,* I.4). The more I feel the body from within, the more attentive I am to the global sensation of the whole body, the more I am able to recognize that I am not the body, but I am essentially the Vision in which the body appears, along with its pleasure and pain. The pain manifests in Awareness, but the Awareness is never in pain, regardless of whether the pain is present or absent. The witness observes the suffering, but does not suffer.

Before recognizing this ever-present peace, I used to practice. After having recognized it, I continue to practice. Daily life and practice, both go on. But they go on with the joy and ease of not taking myself to be someone seeking to control phenomena, not thinking that I am accomplishing some kind of "transformation." And if any change takes place, it will, in any case, appear in Awareness. And then, it will disappear, just as it appeared. Thus the only "concern" is about presence to the present moment, unconditional openness to phenomena, without expectations, just for the joy of being present. I practice, I read, I eat, and I live my life, with the lightness and bliss of one who has let go of a useless burden. Let go, especially of the one who holds on to everything.

Nothing changes, and nothing has changed. Except maybe the fact that, formerly, I used to practice to obtain something, and now, I practice in order to celebrate the life that makes my heart beat, that makes the plants grow and the birds sing; the life without which the love of friendship and relationships would not exist. The joy of being is not the result of a particular phenomenon; it is inherent to the space of Awareness in which the phenomenon manifests. This recognition is in itself a celebration, an offering, completeness, and the pure joy of being; it is love and compassion. It is free, and it is the promise of a never-ending vacation.

Regardless of the season, the moment, or the situation, one always has the opportunity to take some time off, to stop what one is doing, rest, and come back to one's self, by taking a moment to listen to the silence in which the mountain, the bustle of the city, the forest, and the rise and fall of the ocean waves appear. Listen to the whispering of the world, admire its beauty, listen to the listening itself. In this openness, the body reacts with ease, naturally responding to the needs of the moment, driven by a mind that is more creative and fluid, operating wisely, no longer controlled by instructions, which are merely baseless reactions imposed by external circumstances and conditioned memories. In this openness full of life, I can realize that, no matter what I do or which action I claim to do, the silent background remains ever-peaceful, like a presence, a Vision, that is always on vacation, naturally free of the trials and tribulations of the person.

Wherever the body goes for a well-deserved rest, and wherever it goes to fulfill an action, Awareness will always support it, and continue to love and embrace it, along with its joys and sorrows, offering peace and calm to those who abandon themselves completely, like they abandon themselves to blissful sleep in which there is neither "me" nor any problem. In this conversion of the gaze, the effacement leaves room for bliss, quietude, and for the deep conviction that no matter what happens, everything will be fine; and that, if the Vision is real, truly recognized, the vacation is necessarily always "good"; and that it is, above all, never-ending.

Suggested Readings

Bonnasse, Pierre. *Yoga Nidra Meditation: The Sleep of the Sages.* Rochester, Vt.: Inner Traditions, 2017.

Chidananda, Swami. *Practical Guide to Yoga.* Rishikesh, India: The Divine Life Society, 1989.

Chinmayananda, Swami. *The Holy Geeta.* Mumbai, India: Central Chinmaya Mission Trust, 1996.

———. *A Manual of Self-Unfoldment.* Mumbai, India: Central Chinmaya Mission Trust, 1993.

Rama, Swami. *Mandukya Upanishad: Enlightenment without God.* Allahabad, India: Himalayan Institute India, 2018.

———. *Path of Fire and Light.* Vol. 2. Honesdale, Penn.: Himalayan International Institute, 1988.

———. *Om the Eternal Witness.* Dehradun, India: Himalayan Institute Hospital Trust, 2007.

———. *Exercises for Joints and Glands: Gentle Movements to Enhance Your Wellbeing.* 2nd edition. Honesdale, Penn.: Himalayan International Institute, 2007.

Sivananda, Swami. *Yoga Asanas.* Rishikesh, India: The Divine Life Society, 2004.

Index

Page numbers in *italics* indicate illustrations.

Books of Related Interest

Yoga Nidra Meditation
The Sleep of the Sages
by Pierre Bonnasse

The Magic Language of the Fourth Way
Awakening the Power of the Word
by Pierre Bonnasse

Breathing as Spiritual Practice
Experiencing the Presence of God
by Will Johnson

Breathing through the Whole Body
The Buddha's Instructions on Integrating Mind, Body, and Breath
by Will Johnson

Yoga of Light
Awaken Chakra Energies through the Triangles of Light
by Pauline Wills

The Yin Yoga Kit
The Practice of Quiet Power
by Biff Mithoefer

The Practice of Nada Yoga
Meditation on the Inner Sacred Sound
by Baird Hersey
Foreword by Sri Krishna Das

Living a Life of Harmony
Seven Guidelines for Cultivating Peace and Kindness
by Darren Cockburn

INNER TRADITIONS • BEAR & COMPANY
P.O. Box 388
Rochester, VT 05767
1-800-246-8648
www.InnerTraditions.com

Or contact your local bookseller